Emergency Care and Safety Institute

CW00326528

Emergency First Aid

Mark Woolcock, Paramedic, ECP
Medical Writer

Alton Thygerson, EdD
Medical Writer

Benjamin Gulli, MD
Medical Editor

Jon R. Krohmer, MD, FACEP
Medical Editor

AAOS
American Academy of Orthopaedic Surgeons

JONES AND BARTLETT PUBLISHERS
Sudbury, Massachusetts
BOSTON TORONTO LONDON SINGAPORE

Jones and Bartlett Publishers
World Headquarters
40 Tall Pine Drive
Sudbury, MA 01776
info@jbpub.com
www.ECSInstitute.org

Jones and Bartlett Publishers Canada
6339 Ormindale Way
Mississauga, Ontario L5V 1J2
Canada

Jones and Bartlett Publishers International
Barb House, Barb Mews
London W6 7PA
United Kingdom

Jones and Bartlett's books and products are available through most bookstores and online booksellers. To contact Jones and Bartlett Publishers directly, call +44 (0) 1278 723553, fax +44 (0) 1278 723554, or visit our website www.jbpub.com.

Production Credits
Chief Executive Officer: Clayton E. Jones
Chief Operating Officer: Donald W. Jones, Jr.
President, Higher Education and Professional Publishing: Robert W. Holland, Jr.
V.P., Sales and Marketing: William J. Kane
V.P., Production and Design: Anne Spencer
V.P., Manufacturing and Inventory Control: Therese Connell
Publisher, Public Safety Group: Kimberly Brophy
Product Manager: Lorna Downing
Senior Production Editor: Susan Schultz
Photo Research Manager/Photographer: Kimberly Potvin
Associate Photo Researcher and Photographer: Christine McKeen
Director of Marketing: Alisha Weisman
Marketing Manager: Brian Rooney
Interior Design: Anne Spencer
Cover Design: Kristin E. Ohlin
Composition: Spoke & Wheel\Jason Miranda
Text Printing and Binding: Imago
Cover Printing: Imago
Cover Photograph: ©Jones and Bartlett Publishers. Photographed by Kimberly Potvin.

The first aid and CPR procedures in this book are based on the most current recommendations of responsible medical sources. The Publisher, however, makes no guarantee as to, and assume no responsibility for, the correctness, sufficiency, or completeness of such information or recommendations. Other or additional safety measures may be required under particular circumstances.

Library of Congress Cataloging-in-Publication Data

Woolcock, Mark.
Emergency first aid / Mark Woolcock, Alton Thygerson ; British Paramedic Association [and] American Academy of Orthopaedic Surgeons, Emergency Care and Safety Institute.
p. ; cm.
ISBN 978-0-7637-6461-6 (pbk.)
1. First aid in illness and injury—Textbooks. 2. Emergency medicine—Textbooks. I. Thygerson, Alton L. II. British Paramedic Association. III. Emergency Care and Safety Institute. IV. Title.
[DNLM: 1. First Aid—methods—Handbooks. 2. Emergencies—Handbooks. WA 39 W913e 2009]
RC86.7.W665 2009
616.02'52—dc22

2008022421

6048

Additional photographic and illustration credits appear on page 150, which constitutes a continuation of the copyright page.

Printed in Thailand
12 11 10 09 08 10 9 8 7 6 5 4 3 2 1

contents

Chapter 1 Background Information 1

Why Is First Aid Important? 1
What Is First Aid? 1
First Aid Supplies 1
First Aid and the Law 2

Chapter 2 Action at an Emergency 8

Recognise the Emergency 8
Decide to Help 8
Call 9-9-9 or 1-1-2 9
Provide Care 11
Disease Transmission 11

Chapter 3 Finding Out What's Wrong 16

Checking the Casualty 16
Initial Check 17
Physical Examination 19
SAMPLE History 24
Recovery Position 25
What to Do Until EMS Arrives 25

Chapter 4 CPR 29

Heart Attack and Cardiac Arrest 29
Chain of Survival 30
Performing CPR 31
Airway Obstruction 39

Chapter 5 Bleeding and Wounds 50

External Bleeding 50
Internal Bleeding 52
Wound Care 55
Wound Infection 56
Special Wounds 57
Dressings and Bandages 57

Chapter 6 Shock 62

Shock 62
Anaphylaxis 63

Chapter 7 Burns 69

Types of Burns 69
Thermal Burns 69
Care for Thermal Burns 71
Chemical Burns 72
Electrical Burns 72

Chapter 8 Head and Spinal Injuries 76

Head Injuries 76
Eye Injuries 79
Nose Injuries 82
Spinal Injuries 83

Chapter 9 Chest, Abdominal, and Pelvic Injuries 89

Chest Injuries 89
Abdominal Injuries 90
Pelvic Injuries 91

Chapter 10 Bone, Joint, and Muscle Injuries 96

Bone Injuries 96
Splinting 99
Joint Injuries 101
RICE Procedure 106
Muscle Injuries 108

Chapter 11 Sudden Illnesses 113

Heart Attack 113
Angina 115
Stroke 115
Breathing Difficulty 115
Fainting 116
Seizures 117
Diabetic Emergencies 118

Chapter 12 Poisoning 124

Poisons 124
Ingested Poisons 124

Glossary 129
Index 135
Image Credits 150

welcome

About the British Paramedic Association (College of Paramedics)

The British Paramedic Association (College of Paramedics) exists to take forward the standards of education and practice for all those involved in providing professional healthcare. It recognises however, that the foundation for good, safe care is based around those people who are faced with everyday accidents and emergencies whilst at home or at work, and the quality of their training and subsequent actions. The British Paramedic Association thus supports this book as being an essential text for anyone undertaking first aid training, allowing them to give safe and effective care.

The aims of this text are to provide safe and evidenced based guidance to anyone encountering a casualty suffering from an acute illness or injury. It is recognised that prompt first aid care, and specifically CPR and AED usage at the earliest juncture, has a positive effect on the health of a casualty. Whether read as a stand alone text, or incorporated into a one-day course, this text will provide you with the most important elements for preserving life, preventing further harm, and promoting recovery.

Visit **www.BritishParamedic.org**

AAOS
AMERICAN ACADEMY OF ORTHOPAEDIC SURGEONS

About the AAOS

The AAOS provides education and practice management services for orthopaedic surgeons and allied health professionals. The AAOS also serves as an advocate for improved patient care and informs the public about the science of orthopaedics. Founded in 1933, the not-for-profit AAOS has grown from a small organization serving less than 500 members to the world's largest medical association of musculoskeletal specialists. The AAOS now serves about 24,000 members internationally.

Welcome to the Emergency Care and Safety Institute

The ECSI is an educational organization created for the purpose of delivering the highest quality training to laypersons and professionals in the areas of First Aid, CPR, AED, Bloodborne Pathogens, and related health and safety fields.

The ECSI offers a wide range of textbooks, instructor and student support materials, and interactive technology, including online courses. Every ECSI textbook is the centre of an integrated teaching and learning system that offers instructor, student, and technology resources to better support instructors and prepare students. The instructor supplements provide practical hands-on, time-saving tools like PowerPoint presentations, DVDs, and web-based distance learning resources. The student supplements are designed to help students retain the most important information and to assist them in preparing for exams. And, a key component to the teaching and learning systems are technology resources that provide interactive exercises and simulations to help students become great emergency responders.

Documents attesting to the ECSI's recognitions of satisfactory course completion will be issued to those who successfully meet the course objectives and criteria for passing the course. Written acknowledgement of a participant's successful course completion is provided in the form of a Course Completion Card, issued by the ECSI.

Visit www.ECSInstitute.org today!

acknowledgments

We would like to thank the following reviewers.

Paul Abdey, Dip IMC Rcs(Ed) SRPara
Kent Police Tactical Medicine Unit
Tactical Training Firearms Unit
Kent Police College
Maidstone
Kent

Dianna Evans, Cert. Ed.
Tactical Medicine and Specialist First Aid Trainer
Bedfordshire Police
Bedfordshire

Dave Halliwell, MSc, Paramedic
Head of Education
South Western Ambulance NHS Trust
Bournemouth
Dorset

Michael Page, BSc (Hons) Cert. Ed. AASI
Member, British Paramedic Association
State Registered Paramedic and Emergency Care Practitioner
Great Western Ambulance Service NHS Trust
Trowbridge
Wiltshire

Andy Pullen
Tactical Medicine and First Aid Trainer
Wiltshire Police
Wiltshire

Paul Savage, Grad Dip Phys MCSP
Sea Survival and First Aid Trainer
The Lifeboat College
Royal National Lifeboat Institute
Poole
Dorset

Susan Warner, Cert. Ed.
Senior Advisor First Aid (Policy and Assurance)
Metropolitan Police Service
London

Throughout this text, the term emergency medical services (EMS) has been used to recognise the modern responses of the ambulance service to 9-9-9 or 1-1-2 calls. Across the United Kingdom, emergency calls will be attended by a range of volunteer, lay, and professional responders who provide prompt and dynamic care. In some cases, this care negates the need for a conventional ambulance response. The combination of paramedics, ambulance technicians, nurse practitioners, first responders, BASICS doctors, and trained fire personnel may all be the first to respond to a 9-9-9 or 1-1-2 call. Thus, EMS is the most descriptive and suitable collective term.

1

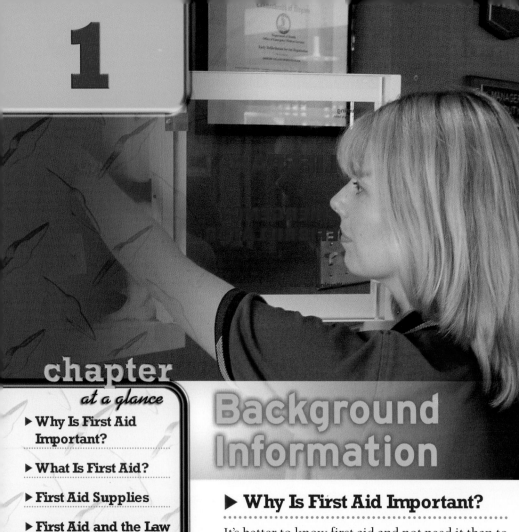

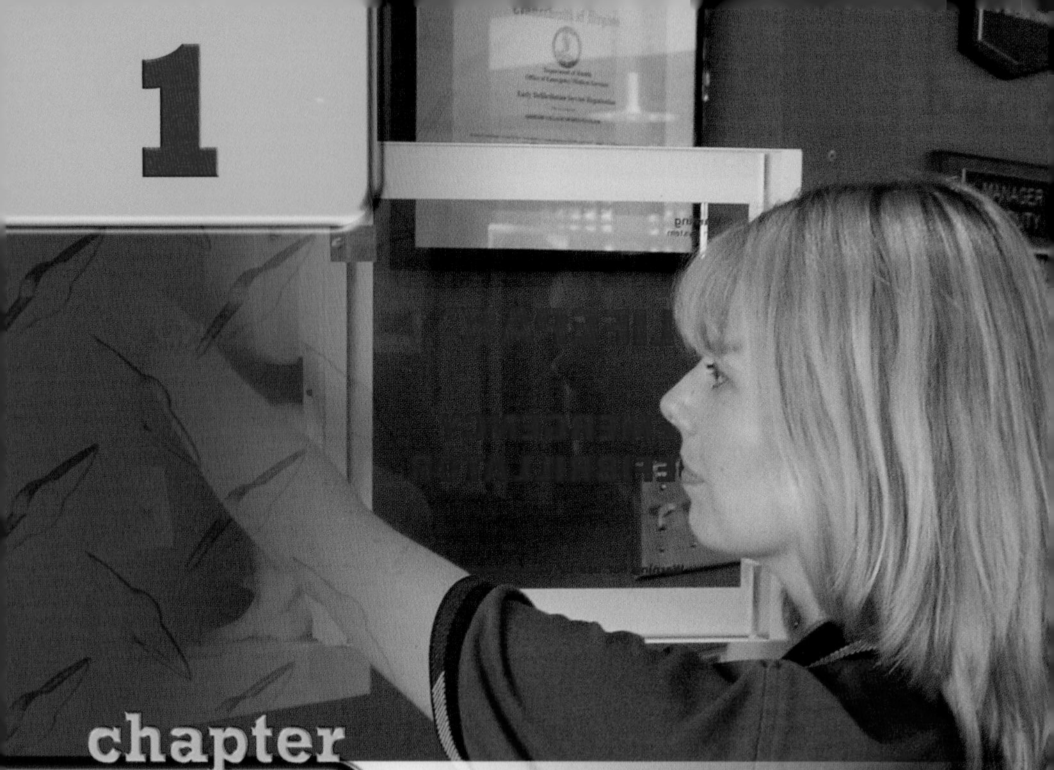

chapter *at a glance*

- Why Is First Aid Important?
- What Is First Aid?
- First Aid Supplies
- First Aid and the Law

Background Information

▶ Why Is First Aid Important?

It's better to know first aid and not need it than to need it and not know it. Everyone should be able to perform first aid, because most people will eventually find themselves in a situation requiring it for another person or for themselves.

▶ What Is First Aid?

First aid is the immediate care given to an injured or suddenly ill person. First aid does not take the place of proper medical care. It consists only of providing temporary assistance until competent medical care, if needed, is obtained or until the chance for recovery without medical care is assured. Most injuries and illnesses do not require medical care. **Figure 1-1** shows the leading causes of nonfatal occupational injuries and illnesses in

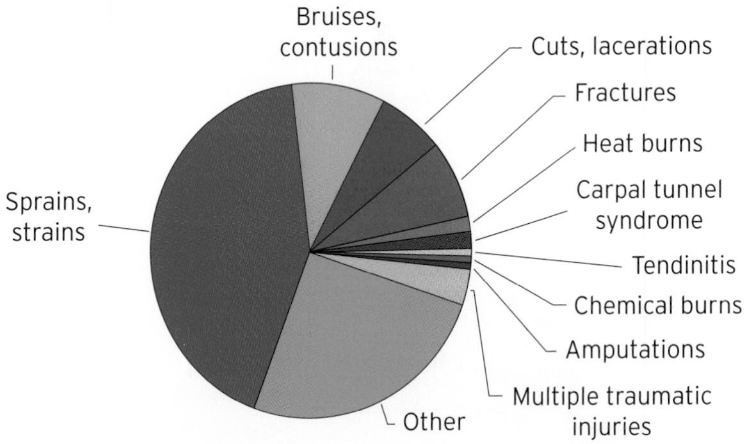

Figure 1-1

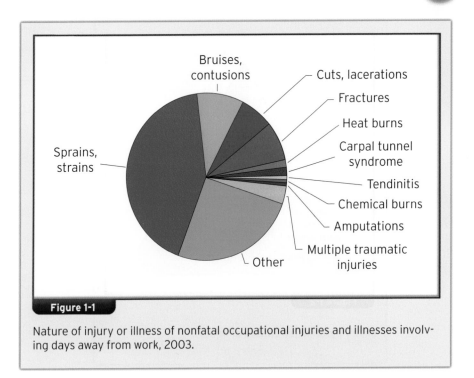

Nature of injury or illness of nonfatal occupational injuries and illnesses involving days away from work, 2003.

the United Kingdom. In the United Kingdom, on average each year, approximately 150,000 people will be injured in some fashion whilst at work, and approximately 200 workers will be fatally injured Figure 1-2.

▶ First Aid Supplies

The supplies in a first aid kit should be customised to include those items likely to be used on a regular basis Figure 1-3. A kit for the home is often different from one for the workplace. A home kit may contain personal medications and a smaller number of items. A workplace kit will need more items (such as bandages) and will not include personal medications. Table 1-1 lists the basic items that should be stocked in a first aid kit for a workplace.

Although a first aid kit may have some medications, such as antihistamines and topical ointments, there may be local requirements that restrict the use of these items by first aiders without prior written approval. For example, teachers, activity leaders, and bus drivers in certain areas may not be able to administer these items to children without specific written permission signed by a child's parent or guardian.

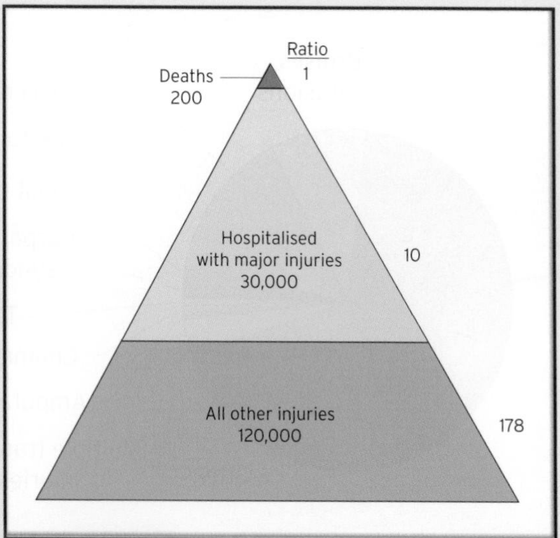

Figure 1-2

Injury pyramid (all causes of injury).

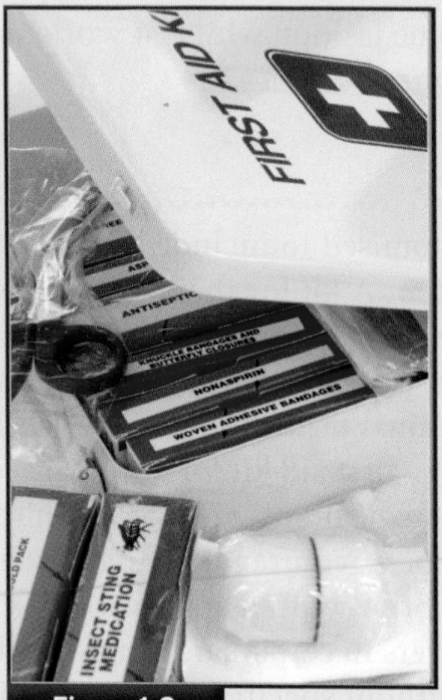

Figure 1-3

Sample first aid kit contents.

▶ First Aid and the Law

Fear of lawsuits has made some people hesitant of becoming involved in emergency situations. First aiders, however, are rarely sued. Below are the legal principles that govern first aid.

The Health and Safety (First Aid) Regulations 1981 are the main source of information regarding first aid in the United Kingdom. To ensure that employees are safe in the workplace, Health and Safety law requires that any employer must assess the level of risk in their place of work and supply an appropriate amount of first aid trained staff and first aid equipment. Employers may choose to send their staff on a First Aid at Work course, which usually lasts for 4 days, or an Emergency First Aid course, which

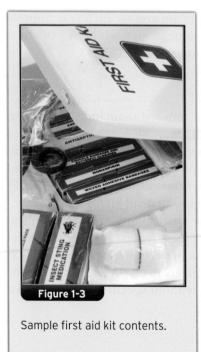

Table 1-1 Sample Workplace First Aid Kit

Equipment	Minimum Quantity
Individually wrapped sterile adhesive dressings (assorted sizes)	20
Sterile eye pads	2
Individually wrapped sterile triangular bandages	4
Safety pins	6
Medium sized non-adhesive/absorbent sterile dressings (12 cm × 12 cm)	6
Large sized non-adhesive/absorbent sterile dressings (18 cm × 18 cm)	6
Sterile conforming roller-gauze bandages	4
Roll of adhesive tape	1
Disposable gloves	2 pairs
Clinical waste-type bag	1
Resuscitation face shield	1

lasts around 1 day. As is always the case, employees must only deliver first aid to the standard for which they have been trained to.

RIDDOR

The Reporting of Injuries, Diseases, and Dangerous Occurrences Regulations 1995 place a legal responsibility on the employer to report to the Health and Safety Executive any of the following occurrences:

- Deaths
- Major injuries
- Accidents that resulted in more than 3 days off work
- Dangerous occurrences
- Diseases

CAUTION

Note the expiry date on every medication. Replace expired medications.

Keep all medications out of the reach of children.

Read and follow all directions for properly using medications.

Good Samaritan Laws

In the United Kingdom, there is no Good Samaritan law, as found in the United States. In essence, this means that there is no legal duty to treat any casualty. This also applies to doctors, nurses, and paramedics. The difference for a health care professional is that whilst they do not have a legal duty to treat, they do have a professional duty.

Duty of Care

Whilst as individuals you are not legally required to provide first aid care, you will still be accountable for your actions and the care you provide. When providing first aid to a casualty, you will have assumed **duty of care**. This ultimately requires you to assess and treat the casualty within the confines of your training and expertise; in essence, you must only do what you have been trained to do.

As long as you act in accordance with the rules and guidelines that you were taught, there should not be any legal liability.

Consent

A first aider must have the **consent** (permission) of a responsive (alert) person before providing care. The casualty may give this permission verbally or with a nod of the head (**expressed consent**). Tell the casualty your name, that you have first aid training, and what you would like to do to help.

When the casualty is unresponsive (motionless), an adult who is mentally incompetent, or a child with a life-threatening condition whose parent or legal guardian is not available, first aiders should assume that **implied consent** is given. This assumes that the casualty (or parent/guardian) would want care provided.

Abandonment

Once you have started first aid, do not leave the casualty until another trained person takes over. Leaving the casualty without help is known as **abandonment**.

Negligence

Negligence occurs when a casualty suffers further injury or harm because the care that was given did not meet the standards expected from a person with similar training in a similar situation. Negligence involves the following:

- Having a duty to act, but either not doing so or doing so incorrectly
- Causing injury and damages

Documentation

Where first aid is provided within the workplace, it will usually be expected that a record of your actions must be kept. Where first aid is provided on the street, it will be impossible to record anything; however, you must ensure that any information is passed onto the EMS provider who may also attend.

When an incident occurs at work, the details must be entered into an accident book, and as a minimum, you should include:

- Date of the intervention
- Name and address of the casualty
- Location of incident
- Type of injury/illness
- Type of treatment given
- Your name and signature

The old adage of 'if you didn't write it down, you cannot prove you did it' is often heard when reviewing records of treatment for casualties, so try to write down every thing you can about the incident.

First Aid Objectives

This chapter covers the following guidelines for First Aid training and will enable the student to be able to:

- Act safely, promptly, and effectively with emergencies at work
- Recognise the contents of a first aid box
- Understand the legal framework
- Maintain simple factual records on the treatment or management of emergencies
- Understand the duties of employers and the legal framework

prep kit

▶ Key Terms

abandonment Failure to continue first aid until relieved by someone with the same or higher level of training.

consent Permission from a casualty to allow the first aider to provide care.

duty of care An individual's responsibility to ensure that any treatment they may provide is in accordance with the training they have taken and within their expertise.

expressed consent Consent explicitly given by a casualty that permits the first aider to provide care.

first aid Immediate care given to an injured or suddenly ill person.

implied consent Consent assumed because the casualty is unresponsive, mentally incompetent, or underage and has no parent or guardian present.

negligence Deviation from the accepted standard of care resulting in further injury to the casualty.

▶ Assessment in Action

You are driving slowly looking for a house number in an unfamiliar residential area. You are attempting to deliver an important package to a customer. You see an elderly woman lying motionless at the bottom of porch stairs outside a house. You see no one else in the neighbourhood, and you are alone. You quickly, but safely, stop your vehicle in front of the casualty's house. As you approach the casualty, you notice that her skin appears bluish.

Directions: Circle Yes if you agree with the statement, and circle No if you disagree.

Yes No **1.** Do you have to stop to help her?

Yes No **2.** You have implied consent to help this person.

Yes No **3.** If she does not respond to your tapping on her shoulders and shouting "Are you OK?" you can leave her and assume that someone else who is more competent or is a family member will arrive shortly to help her.

Yes No **4.** You decide to help. Without examining the casualty you quickly straighten her legs, which suddenly causes a bone to protrude through the skin. Would this increase the likelihood of being sued?

Answers: **1.** No; **1.** Yes; **3.** No; **4.** Yes

▶ Check Your Knowledge

Directions: Circle Yes if you agree with the statement, and circle No if you disagree.

Yes No **1.** Because an ambulance can arrive within minutes in most locations, most people do not need to learn first aid.

Yes No **2.** Correct first aid can mean the difference between life and death.

Yes No **3.** During your lifetime, you are likely to encounter many life-threatening emergencies.

Yes No **4.** All injured casualties need medical care.

Yes No **5.** Before giving first aid, you must get consent (permission) from an alert, competent adult casualty.

Yes No **6.** If you ask an injured adult if you can help, and she says "No," you can ignore her and proceed to provide care.

Yes No **7.** People who are designated as first aiders by their employer must give first aid to injured employees while on the job.

Yes No **8.** First aiders who help injured casualties are rarely sued.

Yes No **9.** Good Samaritan laws will protect you if you carry out a procedure you are not trained to do.

Yes No **10.** You are required to provide first aid to any injured or suddenly ill person you encounter.

Answers: **1.** No; **2.** Yes; **3.** No; **4.** No; **5.** Yes; **6.** No; **7.** Yes; **8.** Yes; **9.** No; **10.** No

2

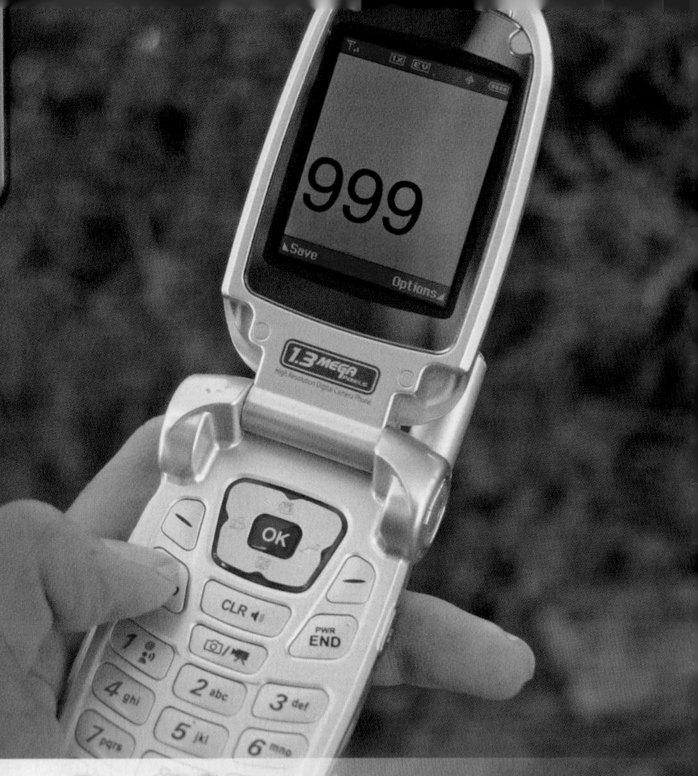

chapter *at a glance*

- ▶ Recognise the Emergency
- ▶ Decide to Help
- ▶ Call 9-9-9 or 1-1-2
- ▶ Provide Care
- ▶ Disease Transmission

Action at an Emergency

▶ Recognise the Emergency

A bystander provides a vital link between medical care and the casualty. Typically it is a bystander who first recognises a situation as an emergency and acts to help the casualty. To help in an emergency, the bystander first has to notice that something is wrong; usually, a person's appearance or behaviour or the surroundings suggest that something unusual has happened.

▶ Decide to Help

At some point, everyone will have to decide whether to help another person. You will be more likely to get involved if you have previously considered the possibility of helping others. Thus, the most important time to make the decision to help is before you ever encounter an emergency.

Size Up the Scene

If you are at the scene of an emergency, take a few seconds to briefly survey the scene, considering three things:

1. *Hazards that could be dangerous to you, the casualties, or bystanders.* Before approaching the casualties, scan the area for immediate dangers (such as oncoming traffic, electrical wires, or an assailant). Always ask yourself: Is the scene safe?
2. *Impression of what happened.* Is it an injury or illness, and is it severe or minor?
3. *How many people are involved.* There may be more than one casualty, so look around and ask about others who might have been involved.

▶ Call 9-9-9 or 1-1-2

Laypeople sometimes make wrong decisions about calling 9-9-9 or 1-1-2. They may delay calling 9-9-9 or 1-1-2 or even bypass emergency medical services (EMS) and transport the seriously ill or injured casualty to hospital in a private vehicle when an ambulance would have been better for the casualty. Some employment situations require that EMS be called rather than having a layperson transport a patient. Fortunately, most injuries and sudden illnesses you encounter will not need more advanced medical care—only first aid. Nevertheless, you should know when to seek medical care.

When to Seek Medical Care

To know when to seek medical care, you must know the difference between a minor injury or illness and a life-threatening one. For example, upper abdominal pain could be indigestion, ulcers, or an early sign of a heart attack. Wheezing may be related to a person's asthma, for which the person can use his or her prescribed inhaler for quick relief, or it can be a severe, life-threatening allergic reaction to a bee sting.

Not every cut needs stitches, nor does every burn require medical care. However, it is always best to err on the side of caution. When a serious situation occurs, call 9-9-9 or 1-1-2 first. Do not call your doctor, the hospital, or a friend, relative, or neighbour for help before you call 9-9-9 or 1-1-2. Calling anyone else first only wastes time. Table 2-1 provides guidance on when to call 9-9-9 or 1-1-2.

How to Call 9-9-9 or 1-1-2

To receive emergency assistance in Britain, you simply dial 9-9-9 and since 2002, the number 1-1-2 allows callers anywhere in the European Union to access the emergency services. These calls are free, irrespective of whether you use a land telephone, call box, or mobile telephone. An operator will put

Table 2-1 When to Call 9-9-9 or 1-1-2

If the answer to any of the following questions is yes, or if you are unsure, call 9-9-9 or 1-1-2 for help.

- Is the casualty's condition life threatening?
- Could the condition get worse and become life threatening on the way to hospital?
- Does the casualty need the skills or equipment of emergency medical technicians or paramedics?
- Would distance or traffic conditions cause a delay in getting to hospital?

The following are specific serious conditions for which 9-9-9 or 1-1-2 should also be called:

- Fainting
- Convulsions
- Chest or abdominal pain or pressure
- Sudden dizziness, weakness, or change in vision
- Difficulty breathing or shortness of breath
- Severe or persistent vomiting
- Sudden, severe pain anywhere in the body
- Suicidal or homicidal feelings
- Bleeding that does not stop after 10 to 15 minutes of pressure
- A gaping wound with edges that do not come together
- Problems with movement or sensation following an injury or severe pain or deformity after injury
- Deep cuts on the hand or face
- Puncture wounds
- The possibility that foreign bodies such as glass or metal have entered a wound
- Most animal bites and all human bites
- Hallucinations and clouding of thoughts
- A stiff neck in association with a fever or a headache
- A bulging or abnormally depressed fontanelle (soft spot) in infants
- Stupor or dazed behaviour accompanying a high fever
- Unequal pupil size, loss of consciousness, blindness, staggering, or repeated vomiting after a head injury
- Spinal injuries
- Severe burns
- Poisoning
- Drug overdose

Source: American College of Emergency Physicians.

you through to any of the emergency services, and you will only be put through to the first one you ask for. When phoning for an ambulance, the call-taker will request some key information:

1. *The location of the emergency.* Give the address, or name of the road, or any landmarks that you can see.
2. *The phone number you are calling from and your name.* This will enable the ambulance control staff to call back should you become disconnected. It may also help to pinpoint the location more accurately.
3. *Casualty's name, condition, and what happened.* You will be asked a series of questions that will help the ambulance controller decide whether extra resources would be needed. One resource will already be activated and making its way toward your location as these questions are being asked.

If you think that another emergency service is required, tell the call-taker this and they will contact either fire or police for you.

Do not hang up! The call-taker will be able to provide you with first aid advice while you are waiting for the first resource to arrive. Also, should the location be difficult to find, it would be possible to get more directions from you. If the call-taker has all the information they require, they may instruct you to hang up, particularly if you need to return to the patient or other helpers.

▶ Provide Care

Often the most critical life support measures are effective only if started immediately by the nearest available person. That person usually will be a bystander.

▶ Disease Transmission

The risk of acquiring an infectious disease while providing first aid is very low. But it can be even lower if you know how to protect yourself against diseases transmitted by blood and air.

Bloodborne Diseases

Some diseases are carried by an infected person's blood (**bloodborne diseases**). Contact with infected blood may result in infection by one of several viruses, such as the following:

- Hepatitis B virus
- Hepatitis C virus
- Human immunodeficiency virus

Hepatitis is a viral infection of the liver. Hepatitis B virus (HBV) and hepatitis C virus (HCV) infections result in long-term liver conditions and can lead to liver cancer. Each is caused by a different virus. A vaccine is available for HBV but not for HCV.

A person infected with human immunodeficiency virus (HIV) can infect others, and those infected with HIV almost always develop acquired immunodeficiency syndrome (AIDS), which is a major cause of death worldwide. No vaccine is available to prevent HIV infection. The best defence against AIDS is to avoid becoming infected.

Airborne Diseases

Diseases transmitted through the air by coughing or sneezing (airborne diseases) include tuberculosis (TB). TB has increased in frequency and is receiving much attention. TB, which is caused by a bacteria, usually settles in the lungs and can be fatal. In most cases, a first aider will not know that a casualty has TB.

Assume that any person with a cough, especially one who is in a nursing home or a shelter, may have TB. Other symptoms include fatigue, weight loss, chest pain, and coughing up blood. If a surgical mask is available, wear it or wrap a handkerchief over your nose and mouth.

Protection

In most cases, you can control the risk of exposure to diseases by wearing personal protective equipment (PPE) and by following some simple procedures. PPE blocks entry of organisms into the body. The most common type of protection involves wearing medical exam gloves **Figure 2-1**. All first aid kits should have several pairs of gloves. Because some rescuers have allergic reactions to latex, latex-free gloves (vinyl or nitrile) should be available.

Protective eyewear and a standard surgical mask may be necessary in some emergencies; first aiders ordinarily will not have or need such equipment. Mouth-to-barrier devices are recommended for cardiopulmonary resuscitation (CPR) **Figure 2-2**.

Always assume that all blood and body fluids are infected. Protect yourself even if blood or body fluids are not visible. At the workplace, PPE must be accessible, and your employer must provide training to help you choose the right PPE for your work.

First aiders can protect themselves and others against diseases by following these steps:

1. Wear appropriate PPE, such as gloves. If they are not available, put your hands in plastic bags or use waterproof material for protection.
2. If you have been trained in the correct procedures, use absorbent barriers to soak up blood or other infectious materials.
3. Clean the spill area with an appropriate disinfecting solution, such as diluted bleach (one quarter cup of bleach in four litres of water).

4. Discard contaminated materials in an appropriate waste disposal container.
5. Wash your hands with soap and water after giving first aid.
6. If the exposure happened at work, report the incident to your supervisor. Otherwise, contact your general practitioner.

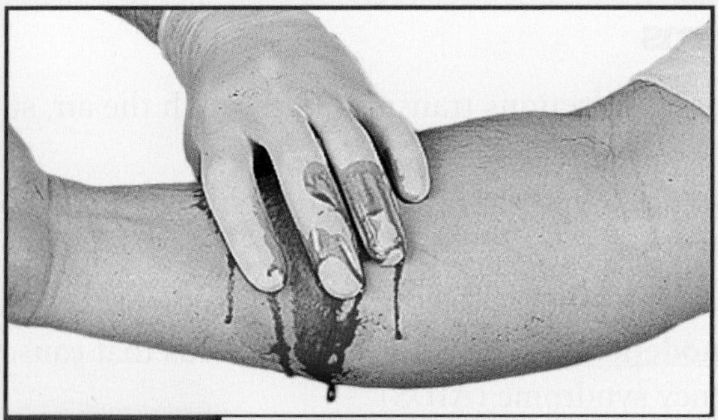

Figure 2-1

Whenever possible, use medical examining gloves as a barrier.

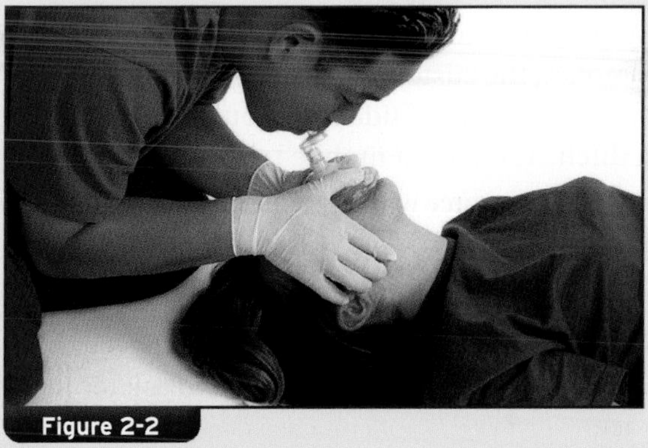

Figure 2-2

Mouth-to-barrier devices are recommended for CPR.

First Aid Objectives

This chapter covers the following guidelines for first aid training and will enable the student to be able to:

- Act safely, promptly, and effectively with emergencies at work
- Recognise the importance of personal hygiene in first aid procedures

prep kit

▶ Key Terms

airborne diseases Infections transmitted through the air, such as tuberculosis.

bloodborne diseases Infections transmitted through the blood, such as HIV or hepatitis B virus.

hepatitis A viral infection of the liver.

human immunodeficiency virus (HIV) The virus that causes acquired immunodeficiency syndrome (AIDS).

personal protective equipment (PPE) Equipment, such as medical examining gloves, used to block the entry of an organism into the body.

tuberculosis (TB) A bacterial disease that usually affects the lungs.

▶ Assessment in Action

You are rushing parts to one of your largest customer's broken machines. Because time is money, the customer is losing a lot for each hour the machine is down. It's beginning to rain. Suddenly, you see a motorcyclist skid off the road and into a ditch. You have a mobile telephone in your car.

Directions: Circle Yes if you agree with the statement, and circle No if you disagree.

Yes No **1.** As you approach the casualty, you should not be concerned about any other possible casualties.

Yes No **2.** This crash scene could be dangerous.

Yes No **3.** You should dial 9-9-9 or 1-1-2 and ask for the ambulance service.

Yes No **4.** Expect to give your name when you call 9-9-9 or 1-1-2.

Yes No **5.** If you do not know the exact address of the emergency, be prepared to give a description of the location as best as you can.

Answers: **1.** No; **2.** Yes; **3.** Yes; **4.** Yes; **5.** Yes

▶ Check Your Knowledge

Directions: Circle Yes if you agree with the statement, and circle No if you disagree.

Yes No 1. A scene survey should be done before giving first aid to an injured casualty.

Yes No 2. For a severely injured casualty, call the casualty's doctor before calling for an ambulance.

Yes No 3. Calling 9-9-9 or 1-1-2 on your mobile telephone is free in Europe.

Yes No 4. First aiders should assume that blood and all body fluids are infectious.

Yes No 5. If you are exposed to blood while on the job, report it to your supervisor, and if off the job, to your personal general practitioner.

Yes No 6. First aid kits should contain medical examining gloves.

Yes No 7. Wash your hands with soap and water after giving first aid.

Yes No 8. Vaccinations are available for both HBV and HCV.

Yes No 9. Medical examining gloves can be made of almost any material as long as they fit the hand well.

Yes No 10. Tuberculosis is a bloodborne disease.

Answers: **1.** Yes; **2.** No; **3.** Yes; **4.** Yes; **5.** Yes; **6.** Yes; **7.** Yes; **8.** No; **9.** No; **10.** No

3

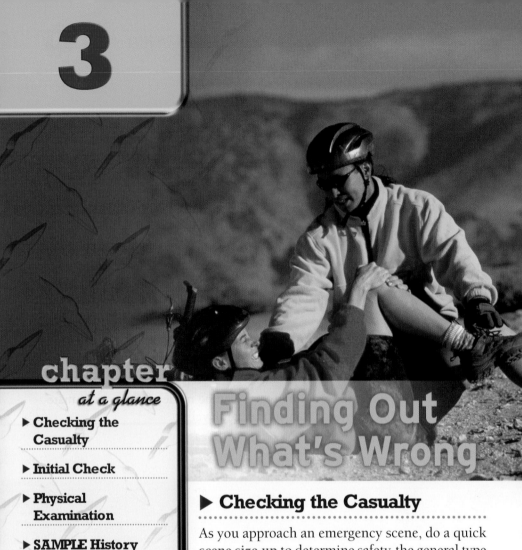

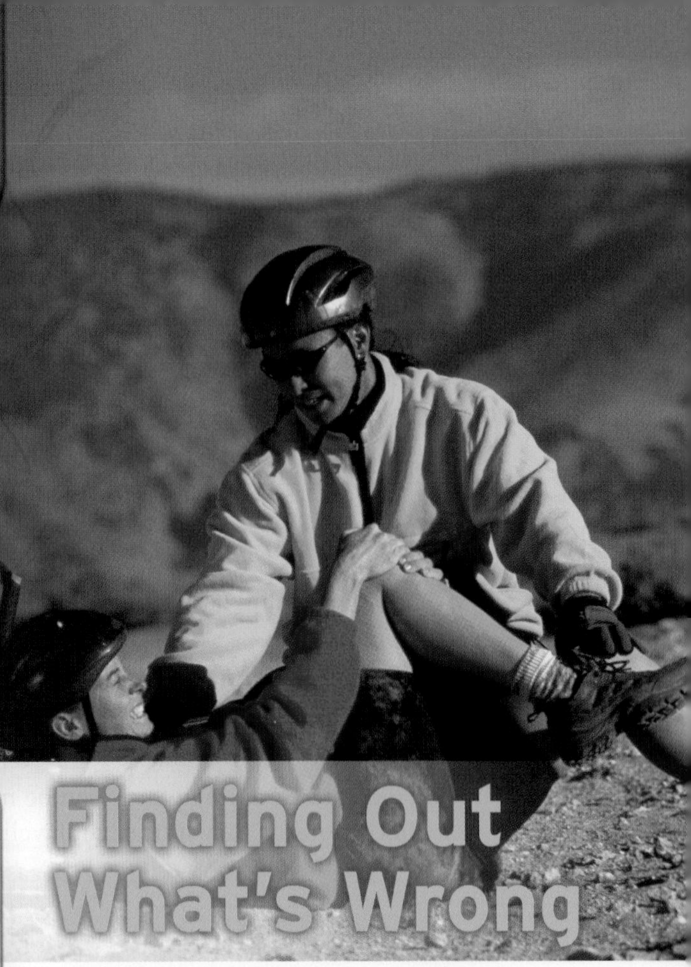

chapter *at a glance*

- Checking the Casualty
- Initial Check
- Physical Examination
- SAMPLE History
- Recovery Position
- What to Do Until EMS Arrives

Finding Out What's Wrong

▶ Checking the Casualty

As you approach an emergency scene, do a quick scene size-up to determine safety, the general type of problem (for example, whether it is an injury or illness and whether it is major or minor), and the number of casualties. If there are two or more casualties, go to the quiet, motionless casualty first.

When you reach the casualty, check to see what is wrong. Identify and correct any immediate life-threatening conditions first.

If there are no immediate threats to life, do a quick physical examination and gather information (history) about the problem.

▶ Initial Check

The initial check determines whether there are life-threatening problems requiring quick care. This step involves checking for the following:

- Responsiveness
- Airway
- Breathing
- Severe bleeding

It will take only seconds to complete this initial check, unless care is required at any point Skill Drill 3-1:

1. *Determine if the casualty is responsive:* Call the casualty in a tone of voice that is loud enough for the casualty to hear. If the casualty does not respond to the sound of your voice, gently tap or shake the casualty's shoulder (**Step 1**).
2. *Ensure that the casualty's airway is open:* In the case of an unresponsive casualty, open the airway by using the head tilt-chin lift manoeuvre (**Step 2**).
3. *Determine if the casualty is breathing:* Look, listen, and feel for signs of breathing (**Step 3**).
4. *Check for any obvious severe bleeding* (Step 4).

Check Responsiveness

If the casualty is alert and talking, then breathing and a heartbeat are present. Ask the casualty his or her name and what happened. If the casualty responds, then the casualty is alert.

If the casualty lies motionless, tap his or her shoulder and ask, "Are you okay?" If there is no response, the casualty is considered unresponsive, and someone should call 9-9-9 or 1-1-2.

Open Airway

In an unresponsive casualty, the airway must be open for breathing. If the casualty is alert and able to answer questions, the airway is open. If a responsive casualty cannot talk or cough forcefully, the airway is probably blocked and must be cleared. In a responsive adult or child casualty, abdominal thrusts can be given to clear a blocked airway. This step is covered in Chapter 4.

In an unresponsive casualty lying face up, open the airway using the head tilt–chin lift method. Once the casualty's airway is open, the initial check can continue.

skill drill

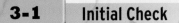

3-1 Initial Check

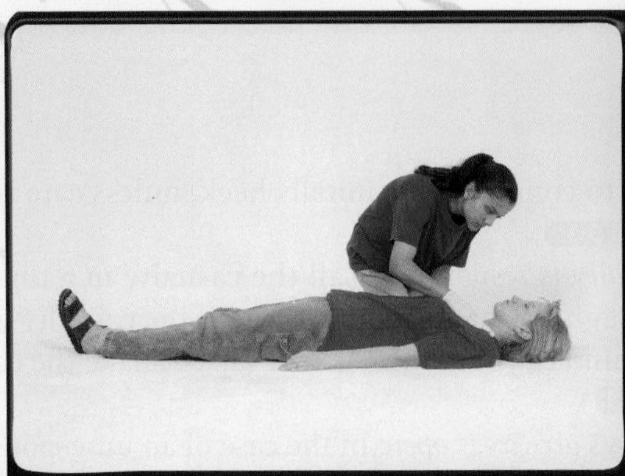

1 Responsive? Tap and shout.

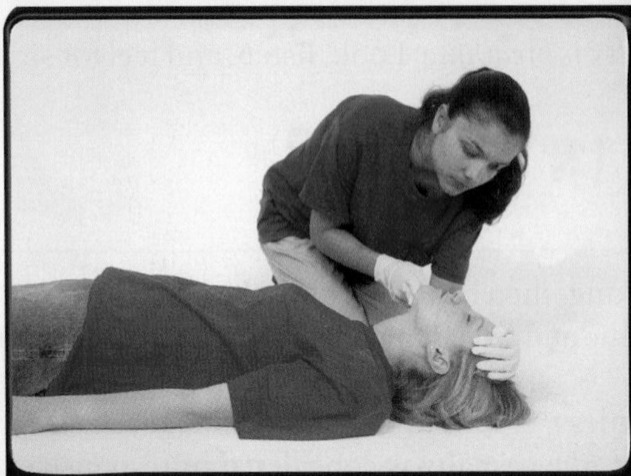

2 Airway open? Perform head tilt-chin lift manoeuvre.

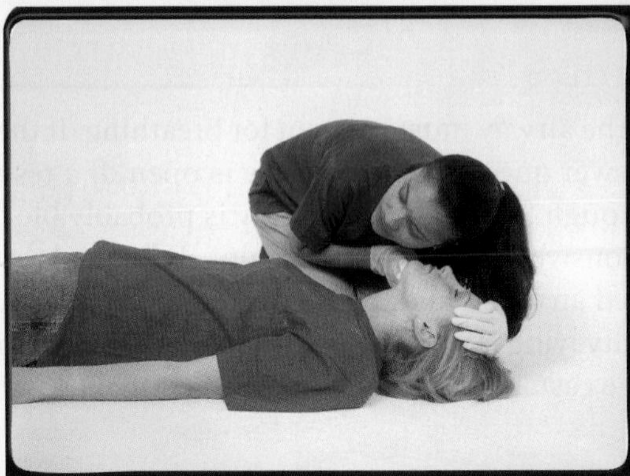

3 Breathing? Look, listen, and feel.

skill drill

3-1 Initial Check (Continued)

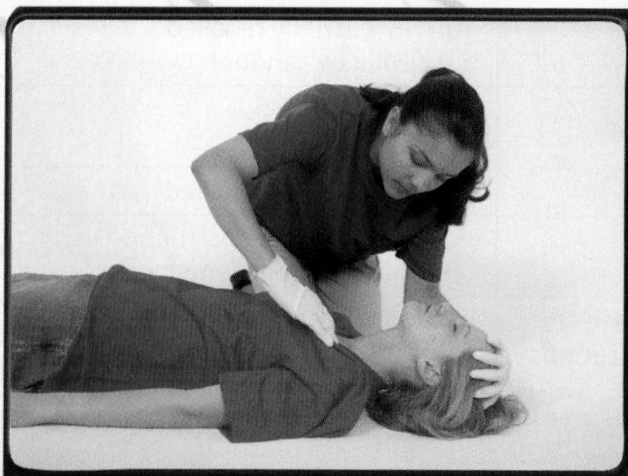

4

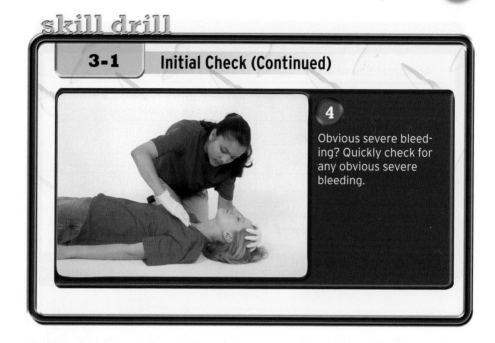

Obvious severe bleeding? Quickly check for any obvious severe bleeding.

Check Breathing

In this step you check to see if the casualty is breathing and, if so, if he or she is having any obvious difficulty breathing. See Table 3-1 for breathing sounds that may indicate a problem.

With the airway of an unresponsive casualty held open, look, listen, and feel for signs of breathing for no more than 10 seconds. Look for the casualty's chest to rise and fall. Listen for breathing sounds. Feel for escaping air on your cheek. If the casualty is not breathing, you must start CPR. See Chapter 4 for CPR procedures.

Check for Severe Bleeding

Check for severe bleeding by quickly scanning for blood up and down the body, for blood-soaked clothing, or for blood collecting on the ground or floor. If you see severe bleeding, control it with pressure. Chapter 5 covers the steps of bleeding control.

▶ Physical Examination

With the initial check complete, and no life-threatening conditions present, perform a quick **physical examination** to gather information about the casualty's condition. During this time you will note the casualty's signs and symptoms.

Table 3-1 Abnormal Breathing Sounds

Abnormal Sound	Possible Causes
Snoring	Airway partially blocked (usually by tongue)
Gurgling (breaths passing through liquid)	Fluids in throat
Crowing (birdlike sound)	Airway partially blocked
Wheezing	Spasm or partial obstruction in bronchi (asthma, emphysema)
Occasional, gasping breaths (known as agonal respirations)	Temporary breathing after the heart has stopped

- Signs = Conditions of the casualty that you can see, feel, hear, or smell
- Symptoms = Things the casualty feels and is able to describe, such as chest pain

For the purpose of this manual, the term signs is used throughout to refer to things you see, feel, hear, and smell, as well as to items the casualty feels and describes.

Check the casualty by looking and feeling for abnormalities. These include deformities, open wounds, tenderness, and swelling. The mnemonic DOTS is helpful for remembering these key signs of a problem.

D **Deformities:** These occur when bones are broken or joints are dislocated, causing an abnormal shape **Figure 3-1**.

O **Open wounds:** These cause a break in the skin and often bleeding **Figure 3-2**.

T **Tenderness:** Sensitivity, discomfort, or pain when touched **Figure 3-3**.

S **Swelling:** The body's response to injury. Fluids accumulate, so the area looks larger than usual **Figure 3-4**.

Since most casualties you encounter will be responsive and able to tell you what is wrong, you can focus your physical examination on the affected area of the body (for example, an injured ankle, painful stomach, or blurry vision).

With casualties who have multiple injuries (for example, from a fall from a height or a motorcycle crash), you may have to check the casualty's entire body to determine the extent of the injuries. In this case, start at the head and proceed down the body looking for signs of problems. If you think the casualty has a possible spinal injury, do not move the casualty. To conduct a physical examination for an injury, follow these steps **Skill Drill 3-2**:

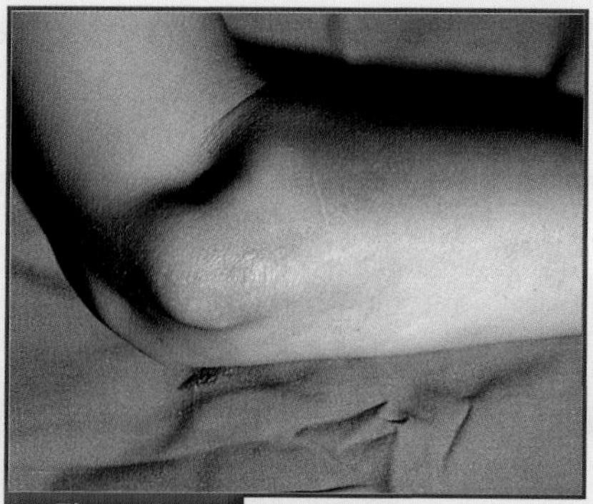

Figure 3-1

D = Deformity.

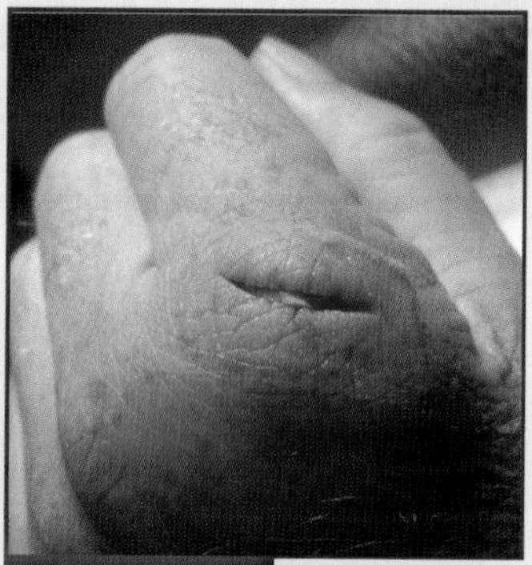

Figure 3-2

O = Open wounds.

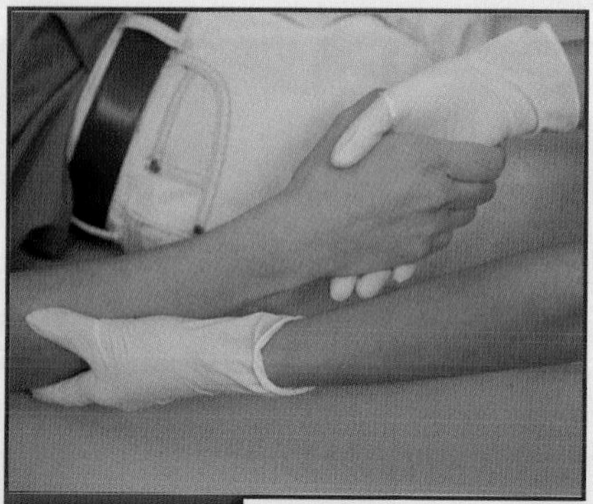

Figure 3-3

T = Tenderness.

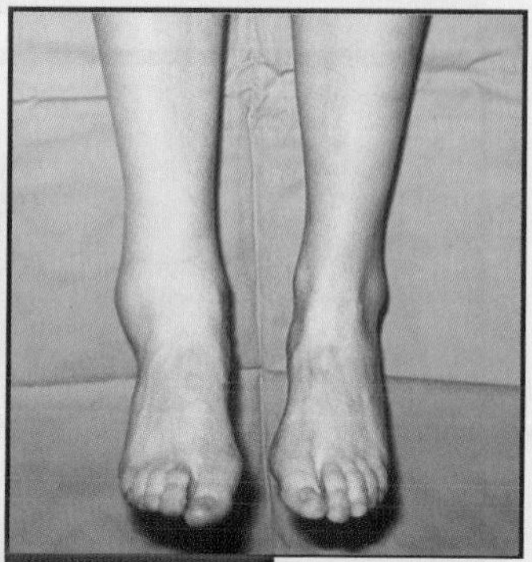

Figure 3-4

S = Swelling.

1. *Head:* Check for DOTS. Compare the pupils—they should be the same size and react to light. Check the ears and nose for clear or blood-tinged fluid. Check the mouth for objects that could block the airway, such as broken teeth (**Step 1**).
2. *Neck:* Check for DOTS. Look for a medical identification necklace or bracelet (**Step 2**).
3. *Chest:* Check for DOTS. Gently squeeze (**Step 3**).
4. *Abdomen:* Check for DOTS. Gently push (**Step 4**).
5. *Pelvis:* Check for DOTS. Gently feel for any movement. Do not apply pressure or "spring" the pelvis (**Step 5**).
6. *Extremities:* Check both arms and legs for DOTS (**Step 6**).
7. *Back:* If no spinal injury is suspected, turn the casualty on his or her side and check for DOTS.

skill drill

3-2 Physical Examination

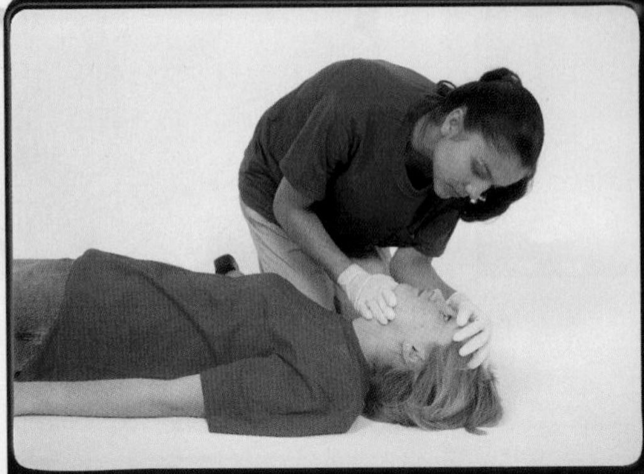

1

Head: Check for DOTS. Compare the pupils-they should be the same size and react to light. Check the ears and nose for clear or blood-tinged fluid. Check the mouth for objects that could block the airway, such as broken teeth.

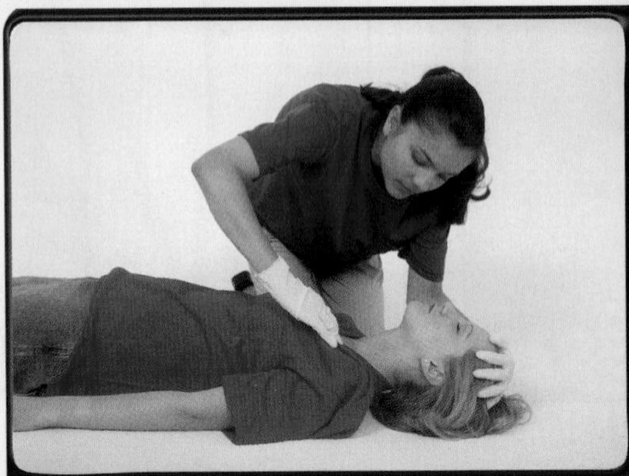

2

Neck: Check for DOTS. Look for a medical identification necklace or bracelet.

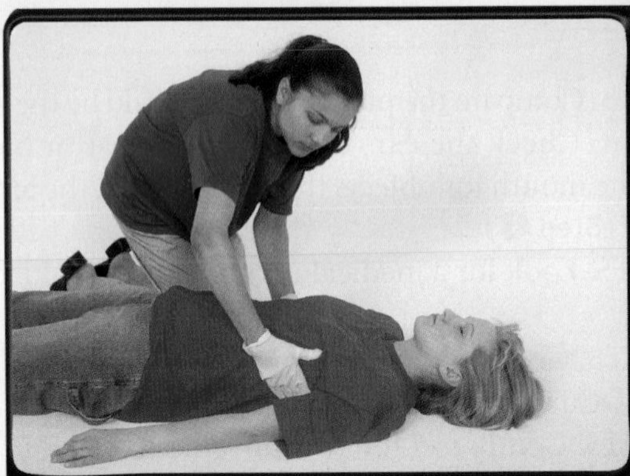

3

Chest: Check for DOTS. Gently squeeze.

skill drill

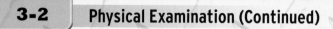

3-2 Physical Examination (Continued)

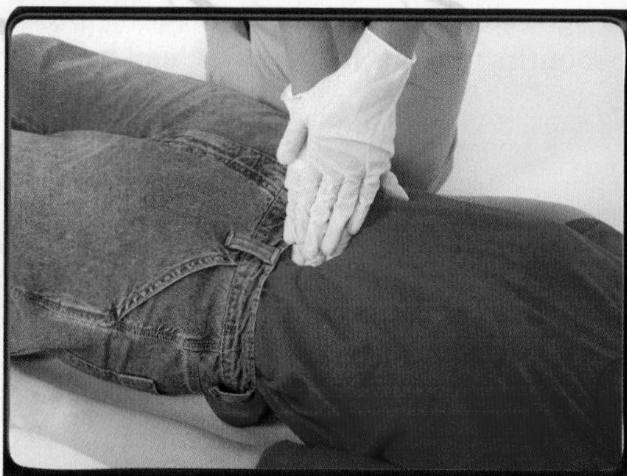

4

Abdomen: Check for DOTS. Gently push.

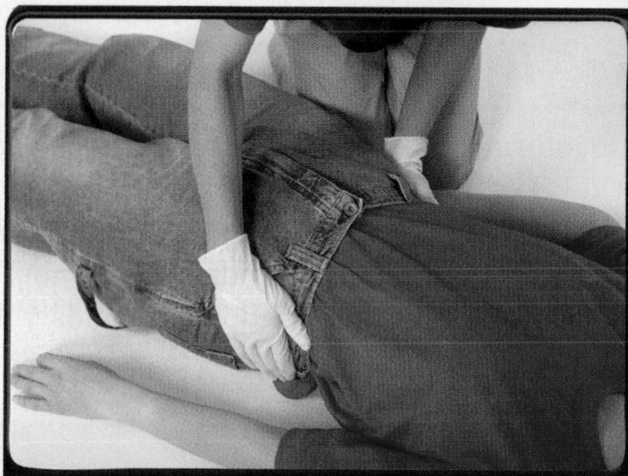

5

Gently feel for any movement. Do not apply pressure.

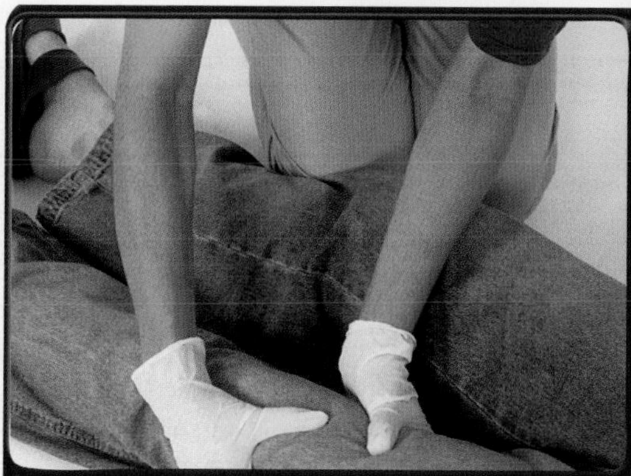

6

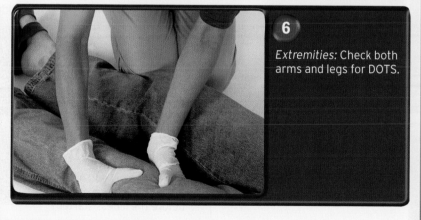

Extremities: Check both arms and legs for DOTS.

While checking the head, check the colour, temperature, and moisture of the skin, which can provide valuable information about the casualty.

Low levels of oxygen in the blood result in the skin and mucous membranes becoming blue or grey (known as cyanosis). This change is usually obvious in the lips and skin of light-skinned individuals. In darkly pigmented persons, it can be seen in the mouth's mucous membranes, nail beds, and inner lining of the eyelids.

A **medical identification tag**, worn as a necklace or as a bracelet, contains the wearer's medical problem(s) and a 24-hour telephone number that offers, in case of an emergency, access to the casualty's medical history plus names of doctors and close relatives. Necklaces and bracelets are durable, instantly recognisable, and less likely than cards to be separated from the casualty in an emergency.

CAUTION

When doing a physical examination:

DO NOT aggravate injuries.

DO NOT move a casualty with a possible spinal injury.

SAMPLE History

An alert casualty may provide information that indicates what is wrong and can indicate the need for first aid. The mnemonic **SAMPLE** helps you remember what information to gather (Table 3-2). If the casualty is unresponsive, you may be able to obtain a history from family, friends, or bystanders. As with the physical examination, gathering this information is secondary if you are dealing with a life-threatening condition.

Table 3-2 SAMPLE History

Description	Questions
S = Signs	"What's wrong?"
A = Allergies	"Are you allergic to anything?"
M = Medications	"Are you taking any medications? What are they for?"
P = Past medical history	"Have you had this problem before? Do you have other medical problems?"
L = Last oral intake	"When did you last eat or drink anything?"
E = Events leading up to the illness or injury	Injury: "How did you get hurt?" Illness: "What were you doing before the illness started?"

Recovery Position

If an unconscious casualty is breathing and has not suffered trauma, the best way to keep the airway open is to place the patient in the recovery position. The recovery position helps keep the casualty's airway open by allowing secretions to drain out of the mouth instead of back into their throat. It also uses gravity to help keep the casualty's tongue and lower jaw from blocking the airway.

To place a casualty in the recover position, carefully roll the patient onto one side as a unit without twisting the body. You will achieve greatest leverage by flexing the casualty's leg that is furthest away and pulling this leg towards yourself. You can use the casualty's hand to help hold his or her head in the proper position. Place the casualty's face on its side so any secretions drain out of the mouth. The head should be in a position similar to the tilted-back position of the head tilt–chin lift manoeuvre Figure 3-5.

What to Do Until EMS Arrives

The initial check, physical examination, and SAMPLE history are done quickly so that injuries and illnesses can be identified and appropriate first aid provided. If possible, record information found during this process and provide this information to arriving EMS personnel. Recheck the casualty's condition every few minutes until EMS personnel arrive. Record any changes in the casualty's condition.

Handover

After arrival of any EMS or health care provider, it is imperative to hand over the casualty properly. This involves introducing the casualty to the newly arrived help and giving a summary of their condition, what you found when you arrived, and most importantly, what treatment or care you have provided.

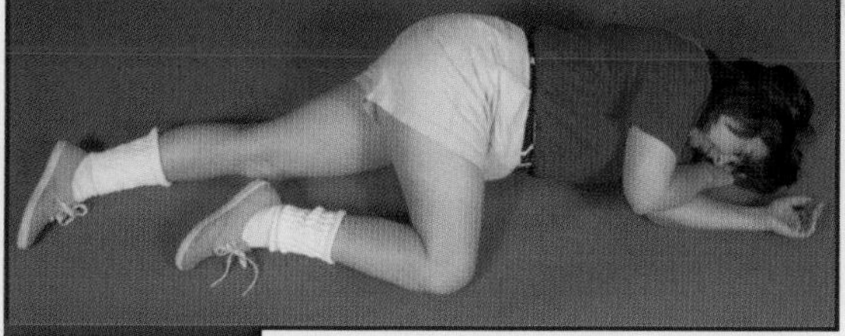

Figure 3-5

Recovery position.

First Aid Objectives

This chapter covers the following guidelines for first aid training and will enable the student to be able to:

- Act safely, promptly, and effectively with emergencies at work
- Recognise a casualty who has a major illness
- Recognise a casualty who has a minor illness

The overall aim of casualty or patient care is to provide a seamless passage from the first person who attends, right through to when the person is discharged or returns home. Make sure your handover is comprehensive, but concise.

prep kit

Key Terms

cyanosis Low levels of oxygen in the blood that result in the skin and mucous membranes becoming blue or grey.

DOTS The mnemonic for remembering key signs of a problem: *Deformities*, *Open wounds*, *Tenderness*, and *Swelling*.

initial check The first step in dealing with an emergency situation; this step determines whether there are life-threatening problems requiring quick care.

medical identification tag A bracelet or necklace that notes the wearer's medical problem(s) and a 24-hour telephone number for emergency access to the casualty's medical history plus names of doctors and close relatives.

physical examination Process of gathering information about the casualty's condition by noting the casualty's signs.

SAMPLE The mnemonic for remembering key information about a patient's history: *Symptoms*, *Allergies*, *Medications*, *Past* medical history, *Last* oral intake, and *Events* leading up to the injury or illness.

scene size-up Quick survey of an emergency scene to determine whether there are life-threatening problems requiring quick care.

Assessment in Action

A colleague calls to report that someone has fallen from a ladder while changing overhead lighting. As a trained first aider, you respond and see people gathered around the casualty. You find the employee lying on the floor motionless. You notice that he wears a medical identification bracelet.

Directions: Circle Yes if you agree with the statement, and circle No if you disagree.

Yes No 1. After confirming that the scene is safe, you next check the medical identification bracelet as a clue for finding out what's wrong.

Yes No 2. If he is unresponsive, you would first look at and feel his legs for a broken bone.

Yes No 3. If he is responsive, you would next gather his health history.

Yes No 4. The physical examination should be started at the casualty's head.

Yes No 5. A medical identification tag lists the casualty's medical problem.

Answers: 1. No; 2. No; 3. No; 4. Yes; 5. Yes

Check Your Knowledge

Directions: Circle Yes if you agree with the statement, and circle No if you disagree.

Yes No **1.** The purpose of an initial check is to find life-threatening conditions.

Yes No **2.** A quiet, motionless casualty may indicate a breathing problem.

Yes No **3.** Most injured casualties require a complete physical examination.

Yes No **4.** For a physical examination, you usually begin at the head and work down the body.

Yes No **5.** If the casualty is not breathing, commence chest compressions once you know help is on the way.

Yes No **6.** The mnemonic DOTS helps in remembering what information to obtain about the casualty's history that may be useful.

Yes No **7.** For all injured and suddenly ill individuals, look for a medical identification tag during a physical examination.

Yes No **8.** The mnemonic SAMPLE can remind you how to examine an area for signs of an injury.

Yes No **9.** If there is more than one casualty, go to the quiet, motionless casualty first.

Yes No **10.** A gurgling sound heard while checking for breathing indicates possible fluid in the throat.

Answers: **1.** Yes; **2.** Yes; **3.** No; **4.** Yes; **5.** Yes; **6.** No; **7.** Yes; **8.** No; **9.** Yes; **10.** Yes

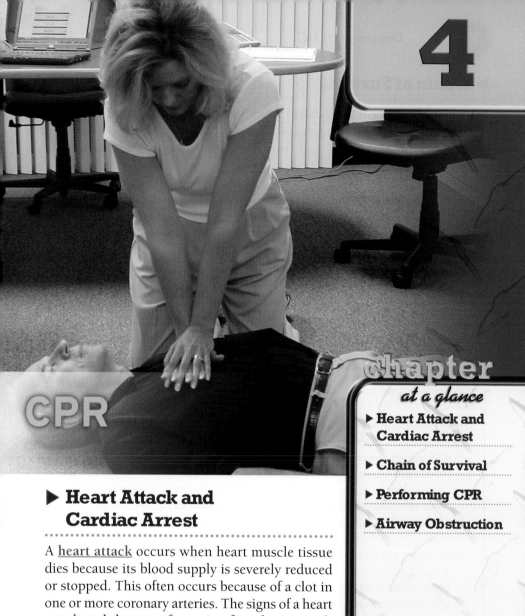

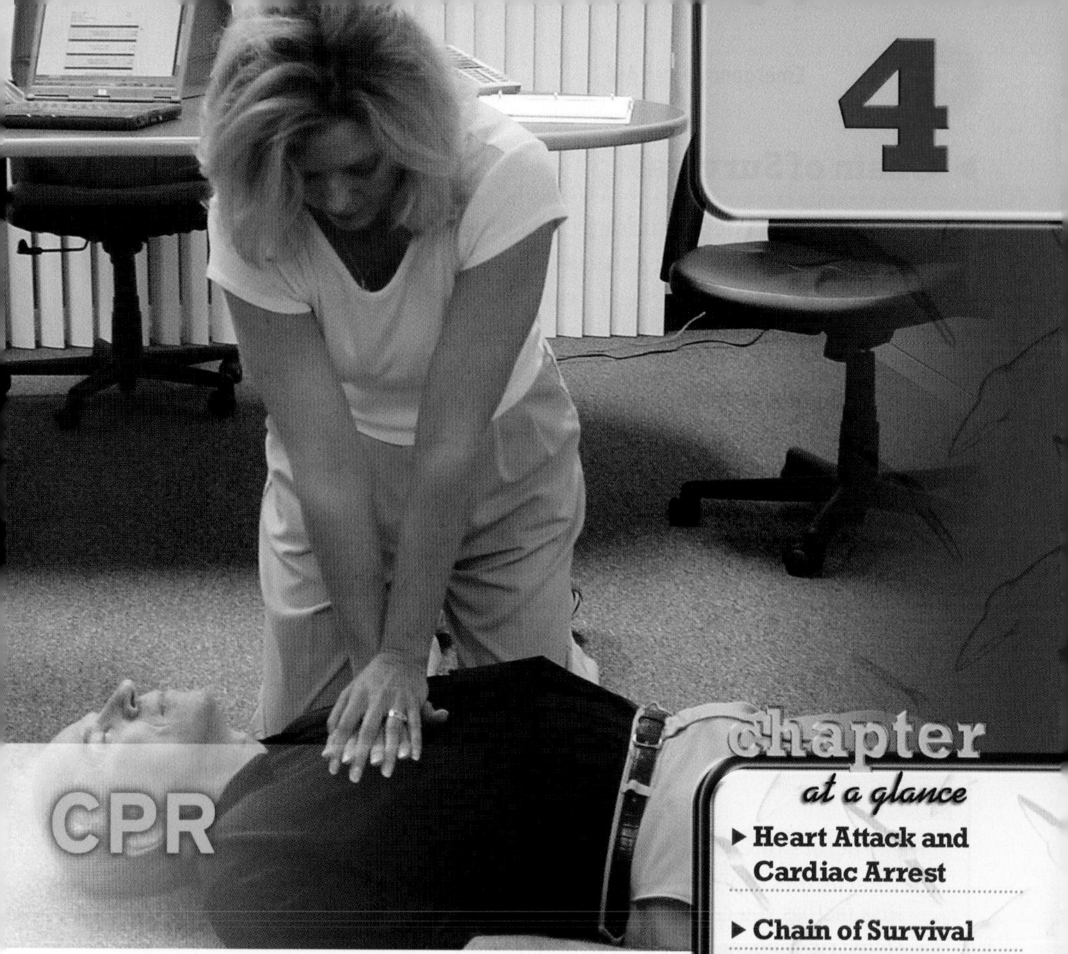

4

CPR

chapter *at a glance*

- Heart Attack and Cardiac Arrest
- Chain of Survival
- Performing CPR
- Airway Obstruction

▶ Heart Attack and Cardiac Arrest

A heart attack occurs when heart muscle tissue dies because its blood supply is severely reduced or stopped. This often occurs because of a clot in one or more coronary arteries. The signs of a heart attack and the steps for caring for a heart attack are discussed in detail in Chapter 11.

If damage to the heart muscle is too severe, the casualty's heart can stop beating—a condition known as cardiac arrest. Sudden cardiac arrest is a leading cause of death in the United Kingdom, affecting about 100,000 people yearly in out-of-hospital locations.

▶ Chain of Survival

Few patients experiencing sudden cardiac arrest outside of a hospital survive unless a rapid sequence of events takes place. The chain of survival is a way of describing the ideal sequence of care that should take place when a cardiac arrest occurs.

The four links in the chain of survival are as follows:

1. *Early access:* Recognising early warning signs and immediately calling 9-9-9 or 1-1-2 to activate emergency medical services (EMS).
2. *Early CPR:* Cardiopulmonary resuscitation (CPR) supplies a minimal amount of blood to the heart and brain. It buys time until a defibrillator and EMS personnel are available.
3. *Early defibrillation:* Administering a shock to the heart can restore the heartbeat in some casualties.
4. *Early advanced care:* Paramedics provide advanced cardiac life support to casualties of sudden cardiac arrest. This includes providing IV fluids, medications, and advanced airway devices.

FYI

Risk Factors of Cardiovascular Disease

Several factors contribute to an increased risk of developing heart disease.

Risk factors you *cannot* change are as follows:

- *Heredity:* Tendencies appear in family lines.
- *Gender:* Men have a greater risk. Even after menopause, when women's death rate from heart disease increases, it is never as high as men's.
- *Age:* Over 80% of those who die from heart disease are 65 years of age or older.

Risk factors you *can* change are as follows:

- *Tobacco smoking:* Smokers have a two to four times greater chance than nonsmokers of developing heart disease.
- *High blood pressure:* This condition increases the heart's workload.
- *High cholesterol:* Too much cholesterol can cause a buildup on the walls of the arteries.
- *Diabetes:* This condition affects blood cholesterol and triglyceride levels.
- *Overweight and obesity:* Excess body fat, especially around the waist, increases the likelihood of developing heart disease. Being overweight affects blood pressure and cholesterol and places an added strain on the heart.
- *Physical inactivity:* Inactive people are more than twice as likely as active people to suffer a heart attack.
- *Stress:* Excessive, long-term stress can create problems in some people.

FYI

Defibrillation

Most adults in cardiac arrest need defibrillation. Early defibrillation is the single most important factor in surviving cardiac arrest.

If any one of these links in the chain is broken (absent), the chance that the casualty will survive is greatly decreased. If all links in the chain are strong, the casualty has the best possible chance of survival.

▶ Performing CPR

When a person's heart stops beating, he or she needs CPR, an AED, and EMS professionals quickly. CPR consists of breathing oxygen into a casualty's lungs and moving blood to the heart and brain by giving chest compressions. CPR techniques are very similar for infants (birth to 1 year), children (1 year to puberty), and adults, with just a few slight variations.

Check for Responsiveness

When the scene is safe, check for responsiveness by tapping the casualty's shoulder and asking if he or she is okay. If the casualty does not respond, ask a bystander to call 9-9-9 or 1-1-2. If you are alone with an adult and a phone is nearby, call 9-9-9 or 1-1-2. If you are alone with an unresponsive child or infant, give five rescue breaths, and if indicated, perform CPR (30:2) for one minute, then call 9-9-9 or 1-1-2.

Open the Airway and Check for Breathing

Place the casualty face up on a hard surface. Before starting CPR, open the casualty's airway and check for normal breathing. Open the airway by tilting the head back and lifting the chin Figure 4-1. This moves the tongue away from the back of the throat, allowing air to enter and escape the lungs. The procedure can be done for injured or uninjured casualties; however, extreme care should be used when injuries to the neck are suspected.

While performing the head tilt–chin lift manoeuvre, check for breathing by placing your ear next to the casualty's mouth. Look at the casualty's chest for rise and fall and listen and feel for other signs of normal breathing for no longer than 10 seconds Figure 4-2.

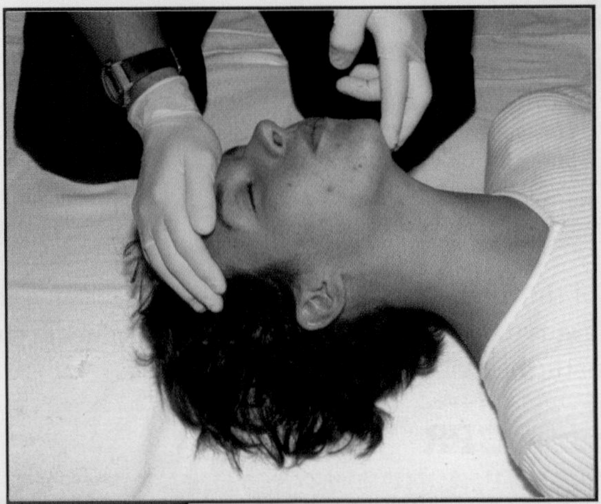

Figure 4-1

The head tilt–chin lift manoeuvre is a simple method for opening the airway.

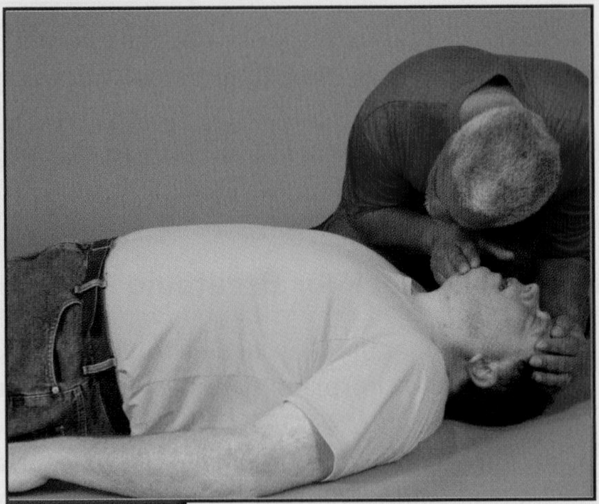

Figure 4-2

Look, listen, and feel for signs of normal breathing.

Chest Compressions

Chest compressions move a minimal amount of blood to the heart and brain. Perform chest compressions with two hands for an adult, one or two hands for a child, and two fingers for an infant. Effective compressions need to be at the correct speed and to the correct depth. Failure to do this properly will greatly reduce the efficacy of the compressions and also the chance of a successful outcome. The chest of an adult should be compressed 4 to 5 cm, and the chest of a child or infant should be compressed one third the depth of the chest. The desired position for adult and child chest compressions is in the centre of the chest between the nipples; for infants, it is just below the nipple line Figure 4-3.

Give 30 compressions at a rate of 100 compressions per minute for adults, children, and infants (a little less than 2 compressions per second).

Combining Chest Compressions with Rescue Breaths

After performing chest compressions, you will need to also start rescue breaths at a ratio of two breaths to every 30 compressions. With the airway open, pinch the casualty's nose and make a tight seal over the casualty's mouth with your mouth. Give one breath lasting 1 second, take a normal breath for yourself, and then give another breath like the first one. Each rescue breath should make the casualty's chest rise. Other methods of rescue breathing are as follows:

- Mouth-to-barrier device
- Mouth-to-nose method
- Mouth-to-stoma method

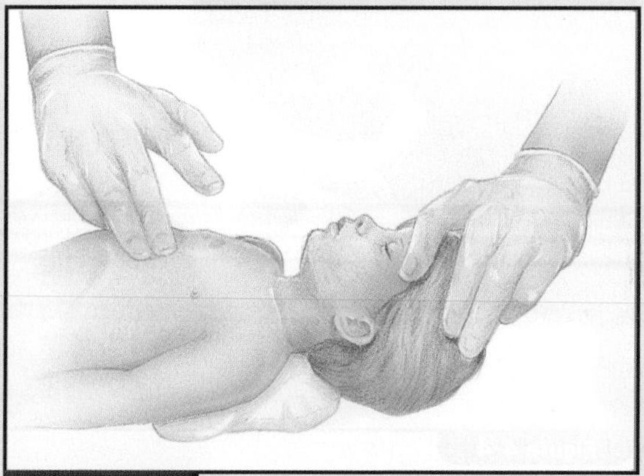

Figure 4-3

Proper hand position for infant CPR.

Mouth-to-Barrier Device A barrier device is placed in the casualty's mouth or over the casualty's mouth and nose as a precaution against infection. There are several different types of barrier devices, and all are easy to use with little modification to the mouth-to-mouth method **Figure 4-4**.

Mouth-to-Nose Method If you cannot open the casualty's mouth, the casualty's mouth is severely injured, or you cannot make a good seal with the casualty's mouth (for example, because there are no teeth), use the mouth-to-nose method. With the head tilted back, push up on the casualty's chin to close the mouth. Make a seal with your mouth over the casualty's nose and provide rescue breaths.

Mouth-to-Stoma Method Some diseases of the vocal cords may result in surgical removal of the larynx. People who have this surgery breathe through a small permanent opening in the neck called a stoma. To perform mouth-to-stoma breathing, close the casualty's mouth and nose and breathe through the opening in the neck.

FYI

Avoiding Stomach Distension

Rescue breaths can cause stomach distension. Minimise this problem by limiting the breaths to the amount needed to make the chest rise. Avoid overinflating the casualty's lungs by just taking a normal breath yourself before breathing into the casualty. Gastric distension can cause regurgitation of stomach contents and complicate care.

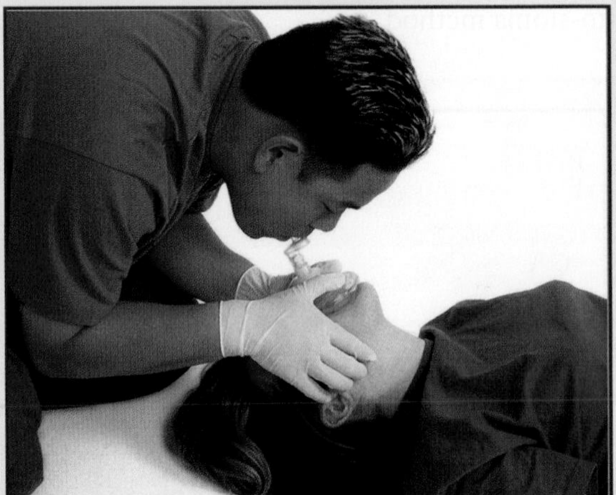

Figure 4-4

Mouth-to-barrier device: mask.

Adult CPR To perform adult CPR, follow the steps in Skill Drill 4-1:

1. Check responsiveness by tapping the casualty and asking, "Are you okay?" If unresponsive, roll the casualty onto his or her back.
2. Have someone call 9-9-9 or 1-1-2 and have someone else retrieve an AED if available.
3. Open the airway using the head tilt–chin lift manoeuvre (Step 1).
4. Check for breathing for no longer than 10 seconds by looking for chest rise and fall and listening and feeling for breathing (Step 2). If the casualty is breathing, place him or her in the recovery position. If the casualty is not breathing, go to the next step.
5. Perform CPR (Step 3).
   - Place the heel of one hand on the centre of the chest between the nipples. Place the other hand on top of the first hand.
   - Depress the chest 4 to 5 cm.
   - Give 30 chest compressions at a rate of about 100 per minute.
   - Open the airway, and give two breaths (1 second each).
6. Continue cycles of 30 chest compressions and two breaths until an AED is available (Step 4), the casualty starts to move, EMS takes over, or you are too tired to continue.

Child CPR To perform CPR on a child, follow the steps in Skill Drill 4-2:

1. Check responsiveness by tapping the casualty and shouting, "Are you okay?" If unresponsive, roll the casualty onto his or her back.
2. Have someone call 9-9-9 or 1-1-2 and have someone else retrieve an AED if available.
3. Open the airway using the head tilt–chin lift manoeuvre (Step 1).
4. Check for breathing for no longer than 10 seconds by looking for chest rise and fall and listening and feeling for breathing (Step 2). If the casualty is breathing, place him or her in the recovery position. If the casualty is not breathing, go to the next step.
5. Give five rescue breaths (1 to 1.5 seconds each), making the chest rise (Step 3). If the first breath does not cause the chest to rise, retilt the head and try the breath again. It is important to give five effective breaths.
6. Perform CPR.
   - Place one hand (Step 4) or two hands on the centre of the chest between the nipples. If two hands are used, place one hand on top of the other as in adult CPR.
   - Depress the chest one third the depth of the chest.
   - Give 30 chest compressions at a rate of about 100 per minute.
   - Open the airway and give two breaths (1 to 1.5 seconds each).
7. Continue cycles of 30 chest compressions and two breaths until an AED is available, the casualty starts to move, EMS takes over, or you are too tired to continue.

skill drill

4-1 Adult CPR

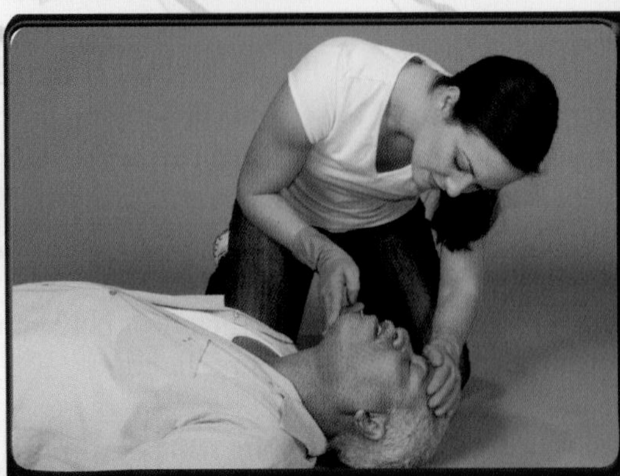

1

Open the airway using the head tilt-chin lift manoeuvre.

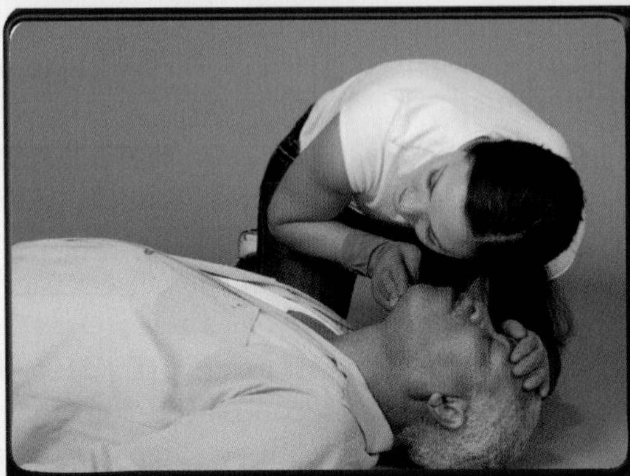

2

Check for breathing for no longer than 10 seconds. If the casualty is breathing, place him or her in the recovery position. If the casualty is not breathing, go to the next step.

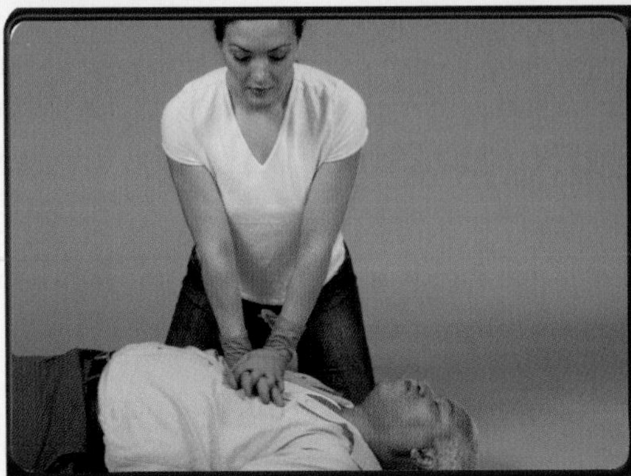

3

Ensure help is on the way. Provide 30 chest compressions (at a rate of 100 per minute) at a depth of 4 to 5 cm.

skill drill

4-1 Adult CPR (Continued)

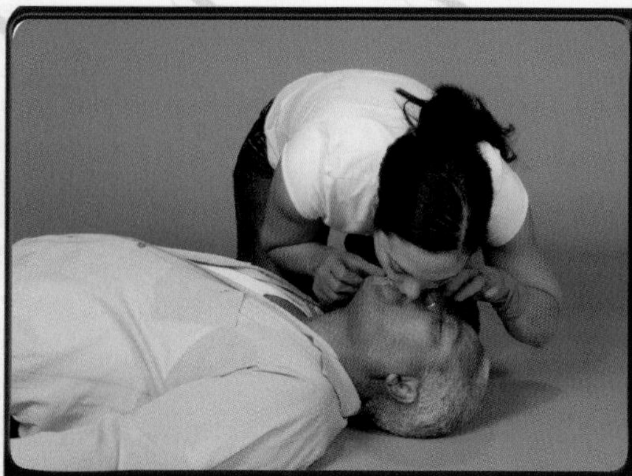

4

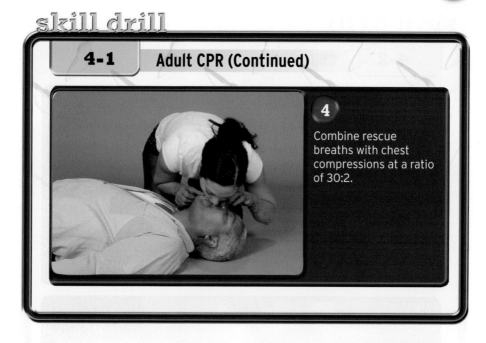

Combine rescue breaths with chest compressions at a ratio of 30:2.

Infant CPR To perform CPR on an infant, follow the steps in Skill Drill 4-3:

1. Check responsiveness by gently stimulating the infant and loudly asking, "Are you okay?" If unresponsive, roll the casualty onto his or her back.
2. Have someone call 9-9-9 or 1-1-2.
3. Open the airway by tilting the head back slightly and lifting the chin (Step 1).
4. Check breathing for no longer than 10 seconds by looking for chest rise and fall and listening and feeling for breathing (Step 2). If the infant is breathing, place him or her in the recovery position. If the infant is not breathing, go on to the next step.
5. Give five rescue breaths (1 to 1.5 seconds each), making the chest rise (Step 3). If the first breath does not cause the chest to rise, retilt the head and try the breath again. It is important to give five effective breaths.
6. Perform CPR (Step 4).
   - Place two fingers on the breastbone just below the nipple line (one finger even with the line).
   - Depress the chest one third the depth of the chest.
   - Give 30 chest compressions at a rate of about 100 per minute.
   - Open the airway and give two breaths (1 to 1.5 seconds each).
7. Continue cycles of 30 chest compressions and two breaths until the infant starts to move, EMS arrives, or you are too tired to continue.

skill drill

4-2 Child CPR

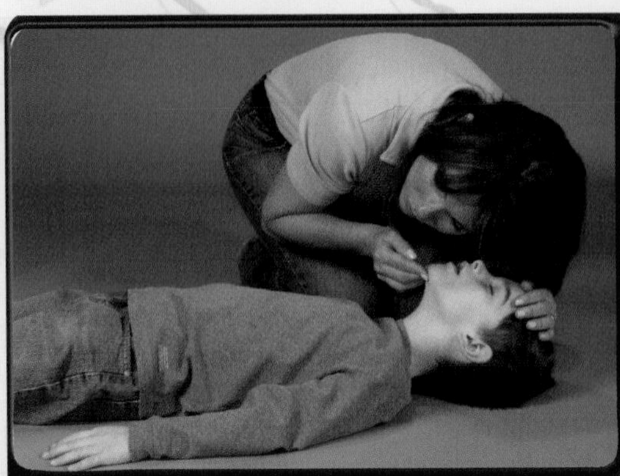

1 Open the airway using the head tilt-chin lift manoeuvre.

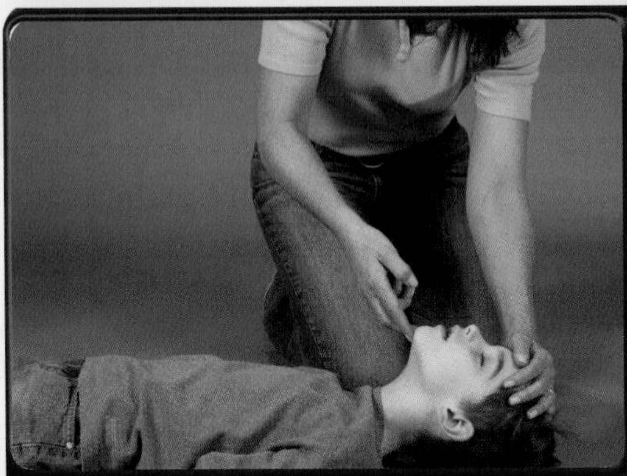

2 Check for breathing for no longer than 10 seconds. If the child is breathing, place him or her in the recovery position. If the child is not breathing, go to the next step.

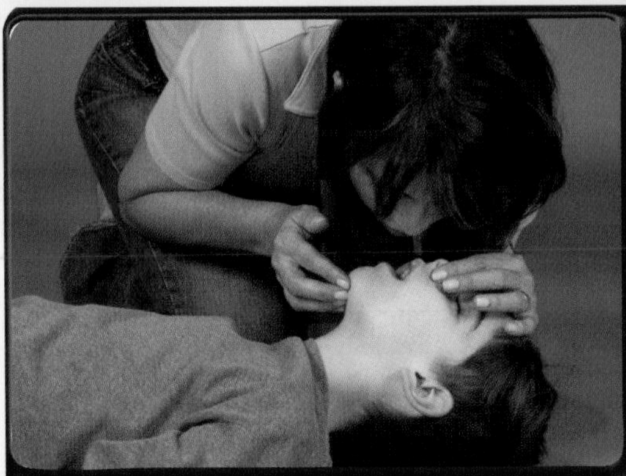

3 Give five initial rescue breaths (1 to 1.5 seconds each). If the first breath does not make the chest rise, retilt the head and try the breath again. If all five breaths made the chest rise, go to the next step.

skill drill

4-2 Child CPR (Continued)

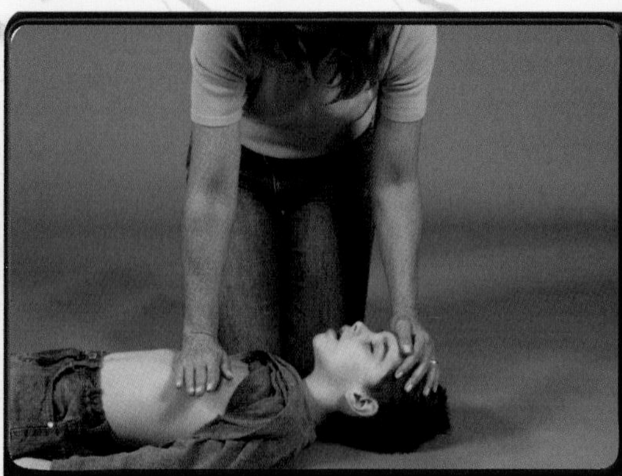

4

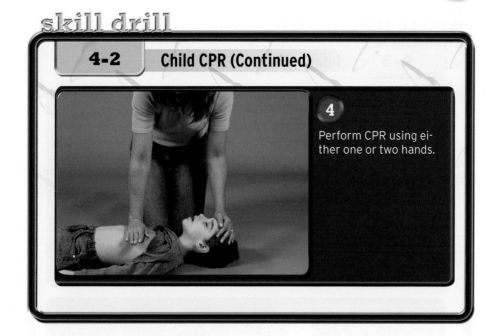

Perform CPR using either one or two hands.

▶ Airway Obstruction

People can choke on all kinds of objects. Foods such as sweets, peanuts, and grapes are major offenders because of their shapes and consistencies. Nonfood choking deaths are often caused by balloons, balls and marbles, toys, and coins inhaled by children and infants.

Recognising Airway Obstruction

An object lodged in the airway can cause a mild or severe airway obstruction. In a mild airway obstruction, good air exchange is present. The casualty is able to make forceful coughing efforts in an attempt to relieve the obstruction. The casualty should be encouraged to cough.

A casualty with a severe airway obstruction will have poor air exchange. The signs of a severe airway obstruction include the following:

- Breathing becoming more difficult
- Weak and ineffective cough
- Inability to speak or breathe
- Skin, fingernail beds, and the inside of the mouth appear bluish grey (indicating cyanosis)

FYI

The Tongue and Airway Obstruction

Airway obstruction in an unresponsive casualty lying on his or her back is usually the result of the tongue relaxing in the back of the mouth, restricting air movement. Opening the airway with the head tilt-chin lift manouvre may be all that is needed to correct this problem.

skill drill

4-3 Infant CPR

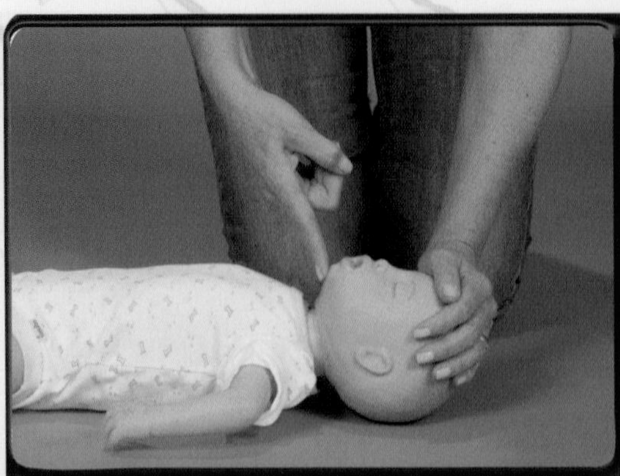

1 Open the airway by tilting the head back slightly and lifting the chin.

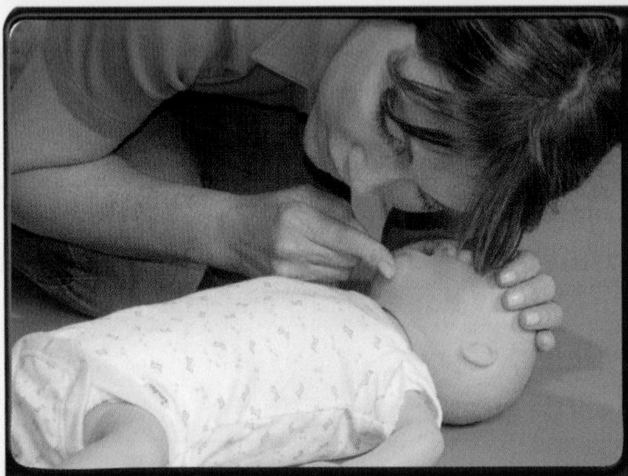

2 Check for breathing for no longer than 10 seconds. If the infant is breathing, place him or her in the recovery position. If the infant is not breathing, go to the next step.

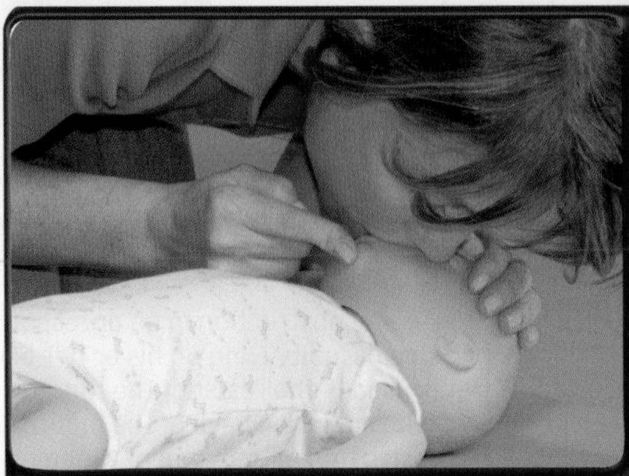

3 Give five initial rescue breaths (1 to 1.5 seconds each). If the first breath does not make the chest rise, retilt the head and try the breath again. If all five breaths make the chest rise, go to the next step.

skill drill

4-3 Infant CPR (Continued)

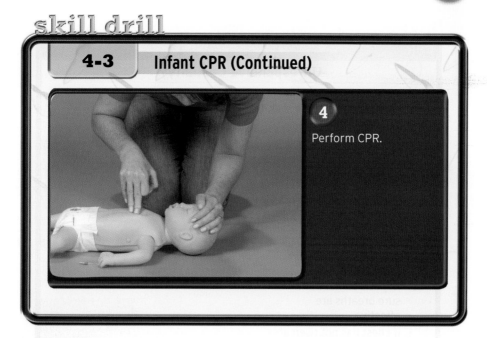

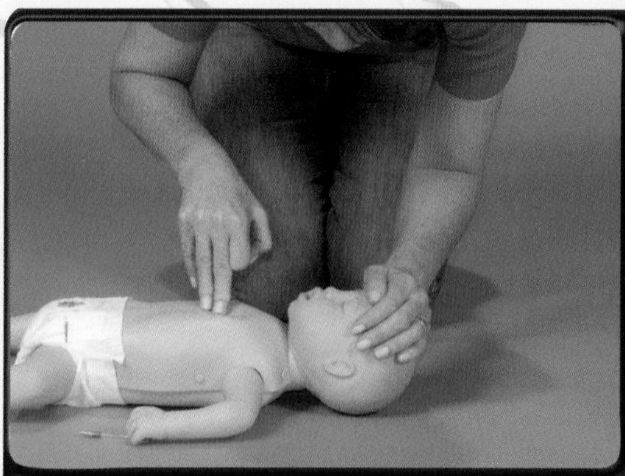

4 Perform CPR.

FYI

Compression-Only CPR

Mouth-to-mouth rescue breathing has a long safety record for casualties and rescuers. But fear of infectious diseases makes some people reluctant to give mouth-to-mouth rescue breaths to strangers.

To avoid the chance that the casualty will not receive any care, compression-only CPR can be considered in these circumstances:

- Rescuer is unwilling or unable to perform mouth-to-mouth rescue breathing.
- Untrained bystander is following ambulance control-assisted CPR instructions.

Choking casualties may clutch their necks to communicate that they are choking. This motion is known as the universal distress signal for choking. The casualty becomes panicked and desperate Figure 4-5.

Caring for Airway Obstruction

For a conscious adult or child with a severe airway obstruction, ask the casualty, "Are you choking?" If the casualty is unable to respond, but nods yes, give the casualty back blows. These are administered by standing slightly behind and to the side of the casualty, and while supporting the casualty to lean forward as far as they can, striking them between the shoulder blades with the heel of your hand. This should be repeated up to five times. If this has

CPR

Unresponsive Casualty?

- Open the airway: Head tilt–chin lift.
- Check for breathing: Look, listen, and feel.

Not Breathing	Breathing
• Have someone call 9-9-9 or 1-1-2 and get an AED if available (for adults and children). • In infants and children, provide 5 breaths. Reposition head to make sure breaths are effective. • If chest has not risen after 5 breaths, commence chest compressions. • Continue to provide single rescuer CPR, looking in the mouth for airway obstructions before giving breaths. • For adults, commence CPR at 30 compressions: 2 breaths, inspecting the airway for obstruction before each breath.	• Place casualty in recovery position.

failed to dislodge the obstruction, administer abdominal thrusts. Move fully around to the back of the casualty and reach around their waist with both arms. Place a fist with the thumb side against the casualty's abdomen, just above the navel. Grab the fist with your other hand and pull sharply inwards and upwards. Repeat up to five times.

If the obstruction is still present, continue to alternate back blows and abdominal thrusts.

For a responsive infant with a severe airway obstruction, give back blows and chest thrusts instead of abdominal thrusts to relieve the obstruction.

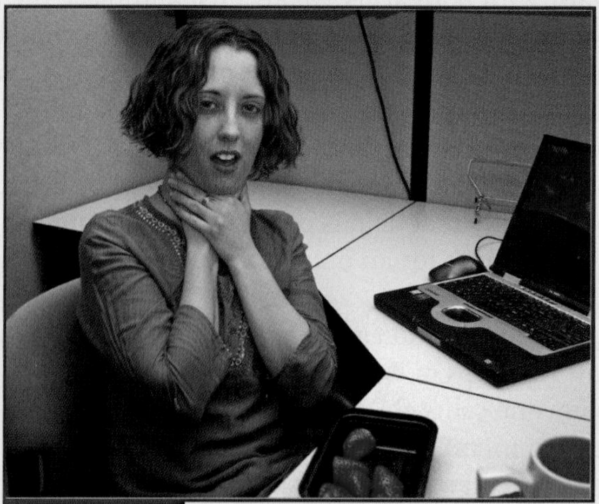

Figure 4-5

The universal sign of choking.

Support the infant's head and neck and lie the infant face down on your forearm, then lower your arm to your leg. Give five back blows between the infant's shoulder blades with the heel of your hand. While supporting the back of the infant's head, roll the infant face up and give five chest thrusts with two fingers on the infant's sternum in the same location used for CPR. Repeat these steps until the object is removed or the infant becomes unresponsive.

If you are caring for an unresponsive, nonbreathing adult casualty with an obstructed airway, you must follow the adult guidelines and perform CPR with a compression to ventilation ratio of 30:2. This should continue until the patient recovers, professional help arrives, or you are too exhausted to continue.

For an unresponsive, nonbreathing infant or child you must open the airway and provide rescue breaths. It is of paramount importance that you assess the effectiveness of each breath by observing for chest rise; if none is seen, you should reposition the head each time before administering the next breath. If after five breaths there is still no response, you should immediately commence chest compressions and follow the CPR guidelines for infants and children.

To relieve airway obstruction in a responsive adult or child who cannot speak, breathe, or cough, follow the steps in **Skill Drill 4-4**:

1. Check casualty for choking by asking, "Are you choking? (**Step 1**).
2. Have someone call 9-9-9 or 1-1-2.
3. Position yourself to the side and slightly behind the casualty. While supporting them to lean forward, strike them between their shoulder blades, up to five times (**Step 2**).

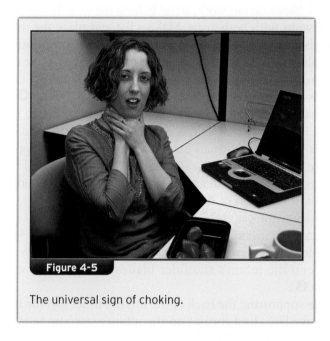

4. If back blows do not work, stand behind the casualty and reach around their waist with both arms. Make a fist and place the thumb side in, just above the navel (**Step 3**), grab the fist with your other hand and pull sharply inwards and upwards, repeating up to five times.
5. Alternate back blows and abdominal thrusts until the obstruction is removed or the casualty becomes unresponsive (**Step 4**).

If the casualty becomes unresponsive, help him or her to the floor and commence CPR. Ensure that help is on the way. Each time you open the airway to give a breath, look for an object in the mouth or throat and, if seen, try to remove it.

To relieve airway obstruction in a responsive infant who cannot cry, breathe, or cough, follow the steps in **Skill Drill 4-5**:

1. Have someone call 9-9-9 or 1-1-2.
2. Support the infant's head and neck and lie the infant face down on your forearm, then lower your arm to your leg. Give five back blows between the infant's shoulder blades with the heel of your hand (**Step 1**).
3. While supporting the back of the infant's head, roll the infant face up and give five chest thrusts on the infant's sternum in the same location used in CPR (**Step 2**).
4. Repeat these steps until the object is removed. If the infant becomes unresponsive, begin CPR. Each time you open the airway to give a breath, look for an object in the mouth or throat and, if the object is seen, remove it.

skill drill

4-4 Airway Obstruction in a Responsive Adult or Child

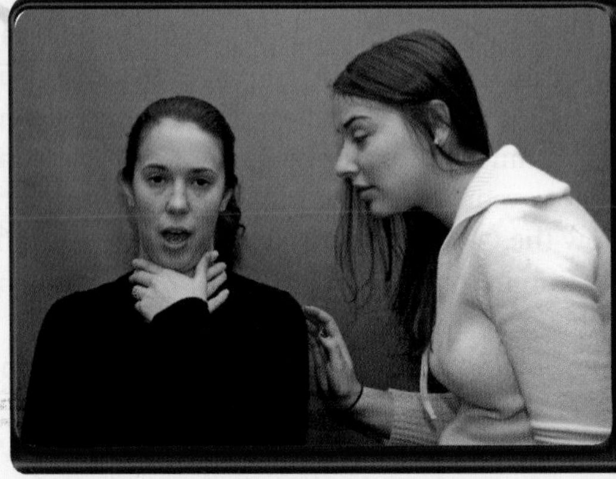

1 Ask the person, "Are you choking?"

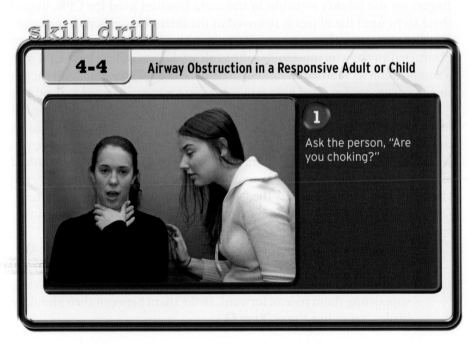

skill drill

4-4 Airway Obstruction in a Responsive Adult or Child

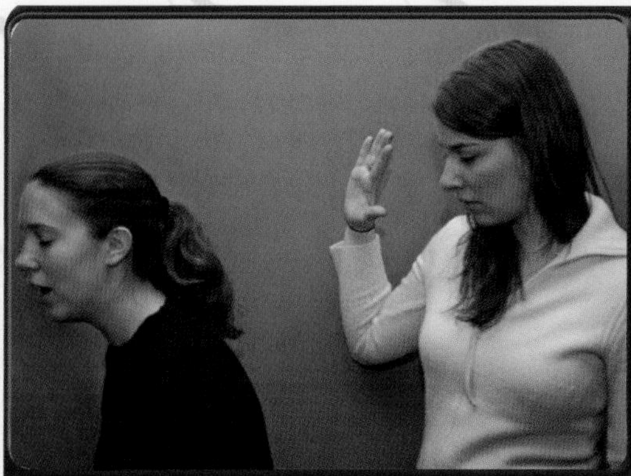

2 Perform five back blows.

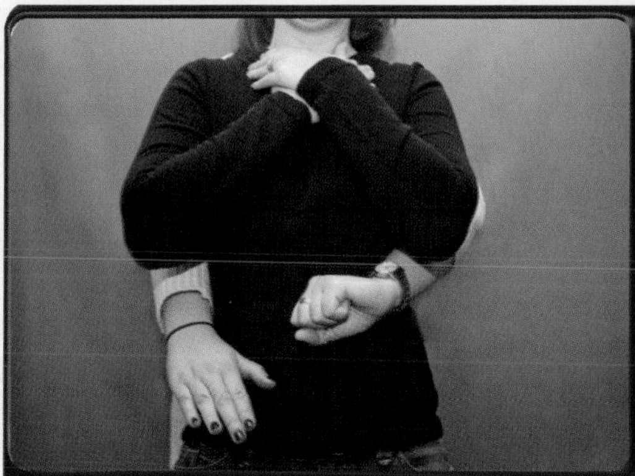

3 Place thumb side of fist just above the navel.

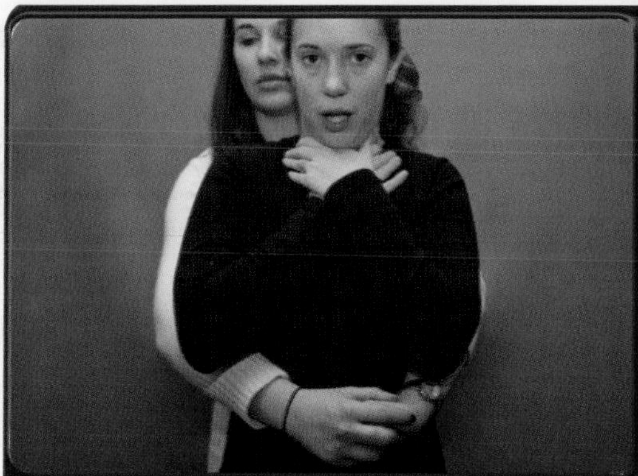

4 Alternate back blows and abdominal thrusts until the obstruction is removed or the casualty becomes unresponsive.

skill drill

4-5 Airway Obstruction in a Responsive Infant

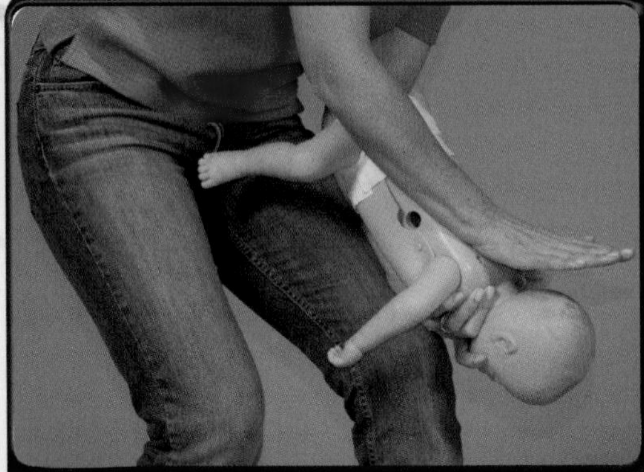

1

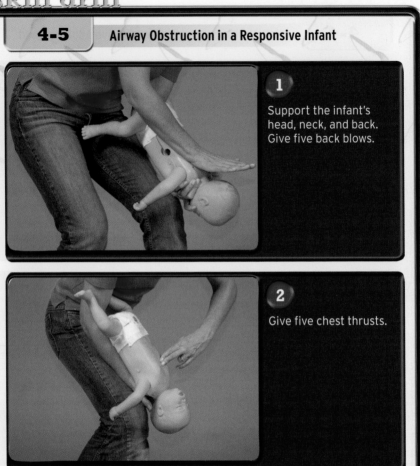

Support the infant's head, neck, and back. Give five back blows.

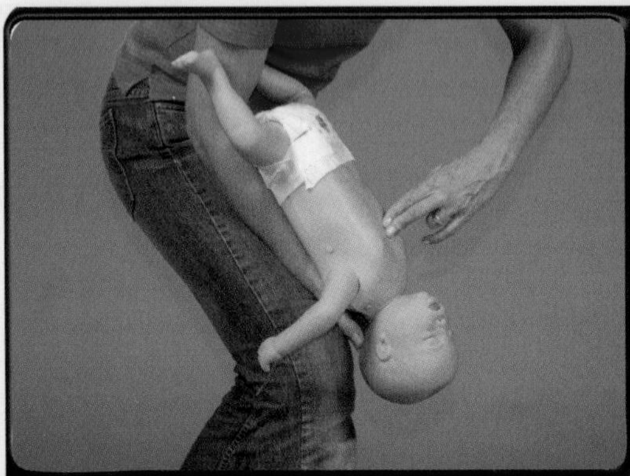

2

Give five chest thrusts.

First Aid Objectives

This chapter covers the following guidelines for First Aid training and will enable the student to be able to:

- Act safely, promptly, and effectively with emergencies at work.
- Recognise the importance of personal hygiene in First Aid procedures.
- Recognise a casualty who has a major illness.
- Deal with a casualty who is unresponsive, choking, or requires cardio-pulmonary resuscitation.

CPR and Airway Obstruction Review

Follow these steps

- Check responsiveness: Tap a shoulder and ask if the casualty is okay. If unresponsive, have someone call 9-9-9 or 1-1-2.
- Open airway: Head tilt–chin lift manoeuvre.
- Check for breathing: Look at the chest to see it rise and fall, and listen and feel for breathing (up to 10 seconds).
- If casualty is breathing but unresponsive, place him or her in the recovery position.
- If an infant or child is not breathing, give five breaths (1½ seconds each).
- If an adult is not breathing, commence chest compressions after getting help.
- In casualties of all ages, perform CPR in cycles of 30 compressions to 2 breaths, at a rate of 100 compressions per minute.

Action	Adult	Child (1 year to puberty)	Infant (<1 year)
1. Breathing methods	Mouth-to-barrier device Mouth-to-mouth Mouth-to-nose Mouth-to-stoma	Mouth-to-barrier device Mouth-to-mouth Mouth-to-nose Mouth-to-stoma	Mouth-to-mouth and nose Mouth-to-barrier device Mouth-to-mouth Mouth-to-nose Mouth-to-stoma
2. Chest compressions			
Locations	On the breastbone, between nipples	On the breastbone, between nipples	On the breastbone, just below nipple line
Method	Two hands: Heel of one hand on chest; other hand on top	One or two hands (depending on size of casualty and rescuer)	Two fingers
Depth	4 to 5 cm	One third the depth of the chest	One third the depth of the chest
Rate	100 per minute	100 per minute	100 per minute
Ratio of chest compressions to breaths	30:2	30:2	30:2
3. When to activate EMS when alone	Immediately after determining casualty is unresponsive	After performing 1 minute of CPR	After performing 1 minute of CPR
4. Use of AED	Yes; deliver one shock as soon as possible, followed immediately by CPR.	Yes; deliver one shock as soon as possible, followed by CPR. Use paediatric pads if available.	No
5. Responsive casualty and airway obstruction	Alternate five back blows followed by five abdominal thrusts repeatedly.	Alternate five back blows followed by five abdominal thrusts repeatedly.	Alternate five back blows followed by five chest thrusts repeatedly.

prep kit

Key Terms

airway obstruction A blockage, often the result of a foreign body, in which air flow to the lungs is reduced or completely blocked.

cardiac arrest Stoppage of the heartbeat.

chain of survival A four-step concept to help improve survival from cardiac arrest: early access, early CPR, early defibrillation, and early advanced care.

chest compressions Depressing the chest and allowing it to return to its normal position as part of CPR.

cardiopulmonary resuscitation (CPR) The act of providing rescue breaths and chest compressions for a casualty in cardiac arrest.

heart attack Death of a part of the heart muscle.

rescue breaths Breathing for a person who is not breathing.

Assessment in Action

You are at a local health club when you overhear someone in the weight room nearby shouting for help. You enter the room and see a person lying motionless on the floor. You quickly confirm that he is unresponsive.

Directions: Circle Yes if you agree with the statement, and circle No if you disagree.

Yes No **1.** The next thing to do is to start chest compressions.

Yes No **2.** The ratio of chest compressions to rescue breaths is 15 to 2.

Yes No **3.** Compression depth for an adult is one third the depth of the chest.

Yes No **4.** Open the airway using the head tilt-chin lift manoeuvre.

Yes No **5.** Continue CPR until an AED becomes available or EMS personnel arrive.

Answers: **1.** No; **2.** No; **3.** No; **4.** Yes; **5.** Yes

Check Your Knowledge

Directions: Circle Yes if you agree with the statement, and circle No if you disagree.

Yes No 1. Take up to 10 seconds when checking for breathing.

Yes No 2. If an adult casualty is unresponsive, the next step is to call 9-9-9 or 1-1-2.

Yes No 3. Tilting the head back and lifting the chin helps move the tongue and open the airway.

Yes No 4. If you determine that an adult casualty is not breathing, begin chest compressions.

Yes No 5. Do not start chest compressions until you have checked for a pulse.

Yes No 6. For all casualties (adult, child, infant) needing CPR, give 30 compressions followed by two breaths.

Yes No 7. Use two fingers when performing CPR on an infant.

Yes No 8. A sign of choking is that the casualty is unable to speak or cough.

Yes No 9. To give abdominal thrusts to a responsive choking casualty, place your fist below the casualty's navel.

Yes No 10. When giving back blows and abdominal thrusts to a responsive adult, alternate five blows and five thrusts until the object is removed or the casualty becomes unresponsive.

Answers: **1.** Yes; **2.** Yes; **3.** Yes; **4.** Yes; **5.** No; **6.** Yes; **7.** Yes; **8.** Yes; **9.** No; **10.** Yes

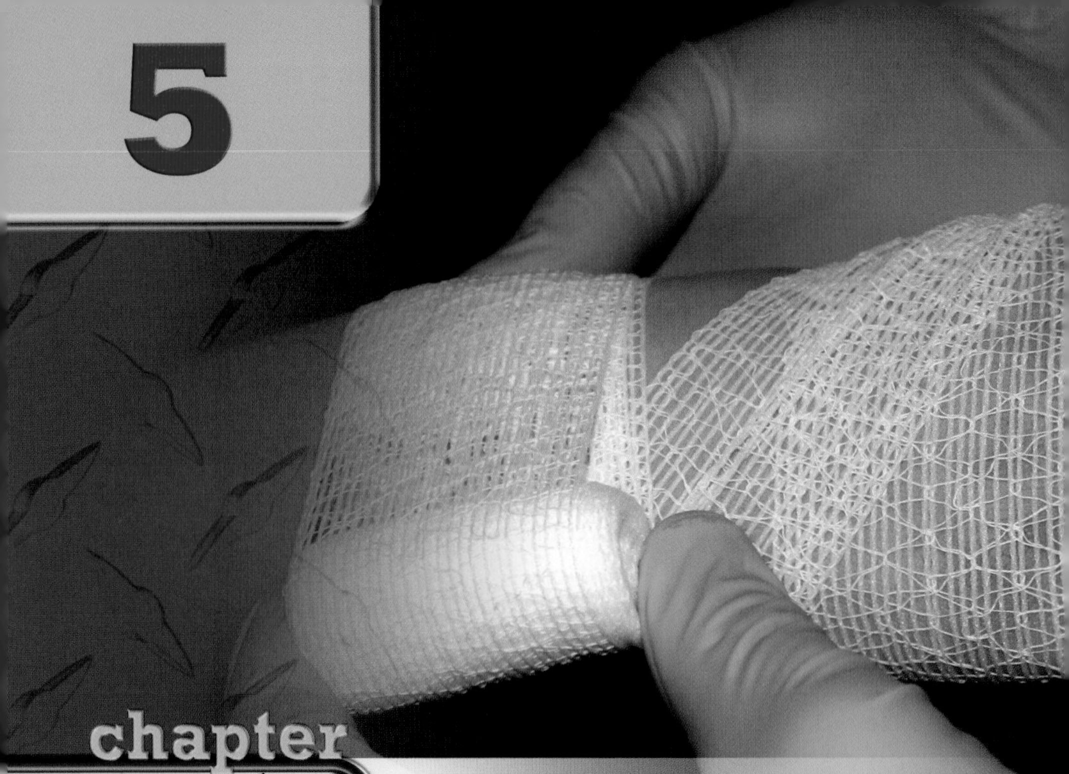

5

chapter *at a glance*

- External Bleeding
- Internal Bleeding
- Wound Care
- Special Wounds
- Dressings and Bandages

Bleeding and Wounds

▶ External Bleeding

External bleeding is the term used when blood can be seen coming from an open wound. The term haemorrhage refers to a large amount of bleeding in a short time.

Recognising External Bleeding

Injuries damage blood vessels and cause bleeding. The three types of bleeding relate to the type of blood vessel that is damaged: capillary, vein, or artery Figure 5-1.

- Capillary bleeding oozes from a wound steadily but slowly. It is the most common type of bleeding and easiest to control.
- Venous bleeding flows steadily. Because it is under less pressure, it does not spurt and is easier to control.

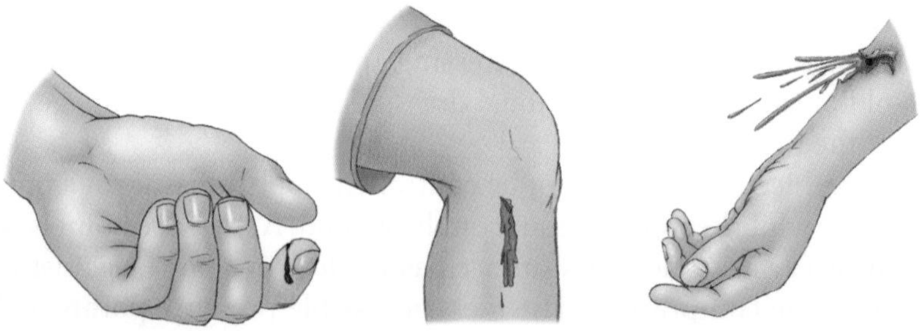

Figure 5-1

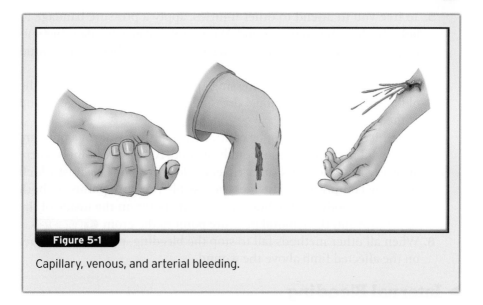

Capillary, venous, and arterial bleeding.

- Arterial bleeding spurts with each heartbeat. The pressure that causes the blood to spurt also makes this type of bleeding difficult to control. This is the most serious type of bleeding because a large amount of blood can be lost in a very short time.

Care for External Bleeding

Care for external bleeding involves controlling the bleeding and protecting the wound from further injury Skill Drill 5-1:

1. Protect yourself against disease by wearing medical examining gloves. If they are not available, use several layers of gauze pads, clean cloths, plastic wrap, a plastic bag, or waterproof material.
2. Expose the wound by removing or cutting the clothing to find the source of the bleeding (**Step 1**).
3. Place a dressing, such as a sterile gauze pad or a clean cloth, over the wound and apply direct pressure with your hand (**Step 2**). This stops most bleeding.
4. If the casualty is bleeding from an arm or leg, elevate the injured area above heart level to reduce blood flow as you continue to apply pressure (**Step 3**).

CAUTION

Once the wound has been cared for, wash your hands with soap and water, even if you used medical examining gloves.

DO NOT use direct pressure on an eye injury, a wound with an embedded object, or a skull fracture.

5. To free you to attend to other injuries, apply a pressure bandage to hold the dressing on the wound. Wrap a roller gauze bandage in a spiral pattern tightly over the dressing and above and below the wound (Step 4).
6. If blood soaks through the dressing and bandage, do not remove the old ones. Apply an additional dressing and pressure bandage on top of the first one.
7. If the bleeding still cannot be controlled, apply pressure at a pressure point while keeping pressure on the wound. A pressure point is where an artery near the skin's surface passes close to a bone, against which it can be compressed. The most accessible pressure points on both sides of the body are the brachial pressure point on the inside of the upper arm and the femoral pressure point in the groin Figure 5-2.
8. When all other methods fail to stop the bleeding, place a tourniquet on the affected limb above the wound.

▶ Internal Bleeding

A closed wound results when a blunt object does not break the skin, but tissue and blood vessels beneath the skin's surface are crushed, causing internal bleeding. In some cases it is easy to detect closed wounds from the bruising that often occurs. In other cases, a closed wound can be difficult to detect but can still be life threatening.

skill drill

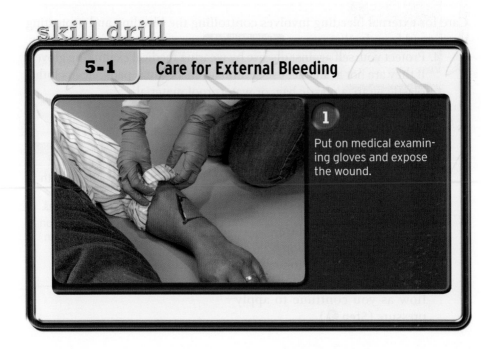

5-1 Care for External Bleeding

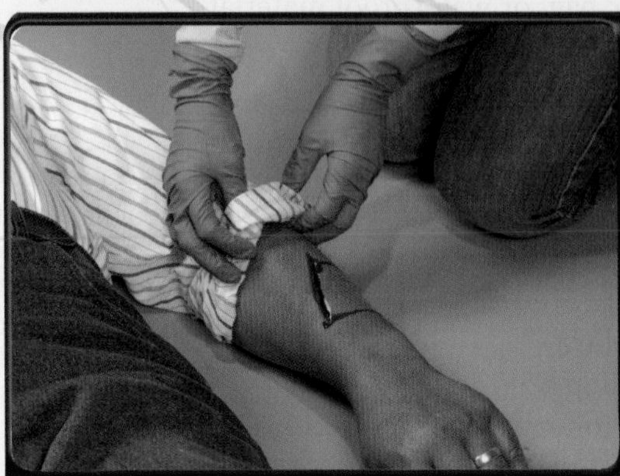

1 Put on medical examining gloves and expose the wound.

skill drill

5-1 Care for External Bleeding (Continued)

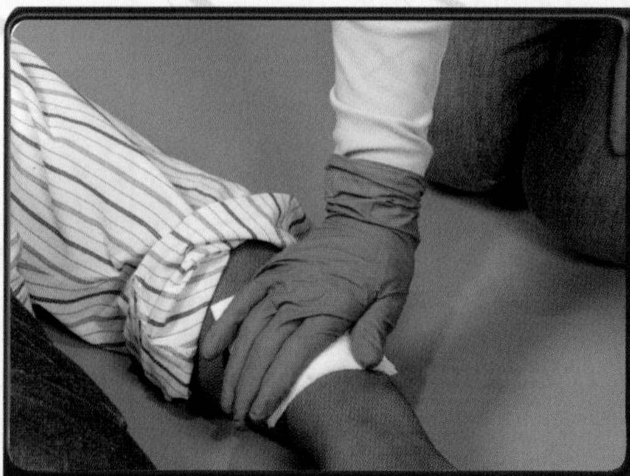

2 Apply direct pressure.

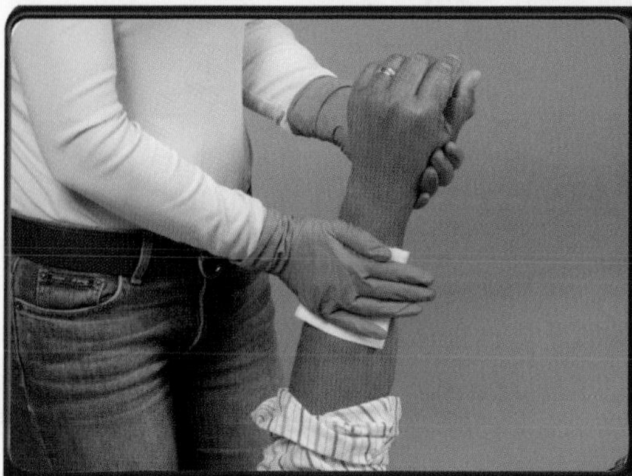

3 Elevate an injured extremity above heart level while keeping pressure on the wound.

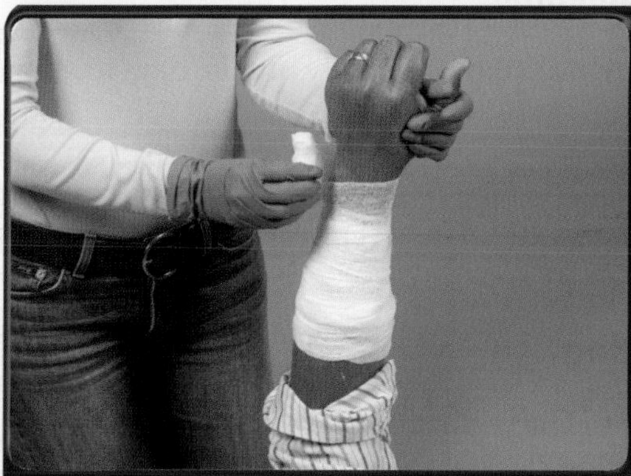

4 Apply a pressure bandage over the dressing and above and below the wound.

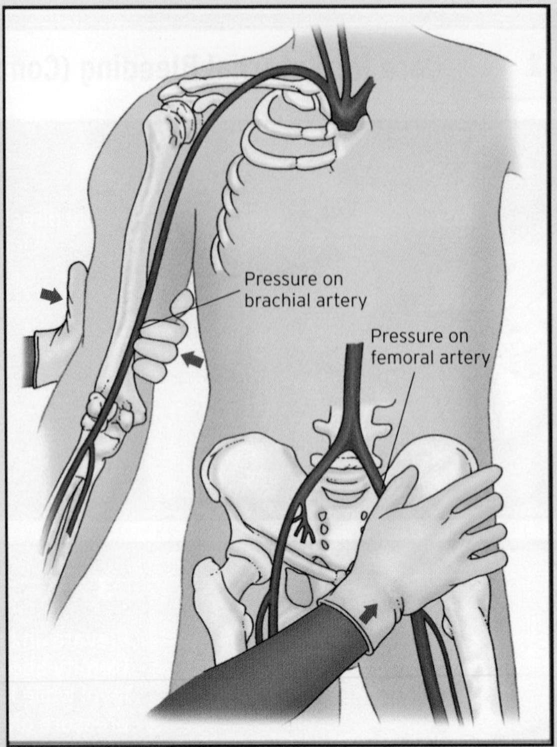

Figure 5-2

Proper hand positions for applying pressure on brachial and femoral arteries.

Recognising Internal Bleeding

The signs of internal bleeding may appear quickly or take days to appear:

- Bruising
- Painful, tender area
- Vomiting or coughing up blood
- Stool that is black or contains bright red blood
- Signs of shock or collapse

Care for Internal Bleeding

For minor internal bleeding (such as a bruise on the leg from bumping into the corner of a table), follow the steps of the RICE procedure:

1. *Rest* the injured area.
2. Apply an *Ice* or cold pack over the injury.
3. *Compress* the injured area by applying an elastic bandage.

4. *Elevate* an injured arm or leg, if it is not broken.

The RICE procedure is presented in more detail in Chapter 10.

To care for serious internal bleeding, follow these steps:

1. Call 9-9-9 or 1-1-2.
2. Care for shock by raising the casualty's legs 25 to 30 cm, and cover the casualty to maintain warmth. See Chapter 6 for more information on shock.
3. If vomiting occurs, roll the casualty onto his or her side to keep the airway clear.
4. Monitor breathing.

CAUTION

DO NOT give a casualty anything to eat or drink. It could cause nausea and vomiting, which could result in aspiration. Food or liquids could cause complications if surgery is needed.

▶ Wound Care

A minor wound should be cleaned to help prevent infection. Wound cleaning usually restarts bleeding by disturbing the clot, but it should be done anyway. For severe bleeding, leave the pressure bandage in place until the casualty can get medical care. To clean a shallow wound:

1. Wash the wound with soap and water.
2. Flush the wound with running water under pressure.
3. Remove small objects that are not flushed out with sterile tweezers.
4. If bleeding restarts, apply direct pressure over the wound.
5. Cover the area with a sterile, absorbent, non-adhesive dressing. Change the dressing and bandage periodically.
6. Seek medical care for a wound with a high risk for infection (such as an animal bite or a puncture).

Tetanus

Tetanus is caused by a bacterium that can produce a powerful poisonous toxin when it enters a wound. The toxin causes contractions of certain muscle groups, particularly in the jaw. There is no known cure for the toxin.

Because of this danger, everyone needs an initial series of vaccinations to defend against the toxin. Nowadays, most people have received immunisation through routine childhood injections, and, providing that these vaccinations are up-to-date, a tetanus booster will only be required for people who are at risk to contracting tetanus because their wound is dirty, was caused by an animal, or because the emergency staff are unsure of the degree of contamination. To be effective, it is recommended that you seek medical attention within 48 hours of being injured.

▶ Special Wounds

This section addresses amputations.

Amputations

The loss of a body part is a devastating injury that requires immediate medical care. To care for an amputation Figure 5-3 :

1. Call 9-9-9 or 1-1-2.
2. Control bleeding.
3. Care for shock.
4. Recover the amputated part and place it in a clean plastic bag or wrap in cling film.
5. Lightly wrap the bagged amputated part in gauze or a clean cloth.
6. Keep the part cool (for example, on an ice or cold pack), but do not freeze.

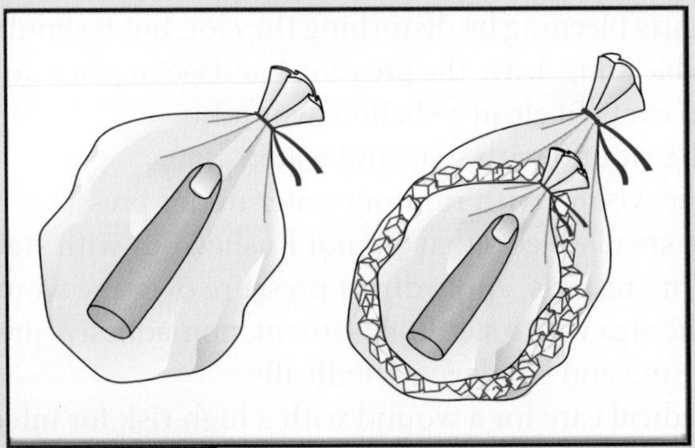

Figure 5-3

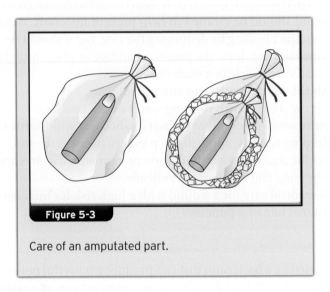

Care of an amputated part.

FYI

Cooling Amputated Parts

Amputated body parts that remain uncooled for more than 6 hours have little chance of survival; 18 hours is probably the maximum time allowable for a part that has been cooled properly. Muscles without blood lose viability within 4 to 6 hours.

▶ Dressings and Bandages

First aid kits include dressings and bandages to be used when controlling bleeding and caring for wounds. A **dressing** is a covering that is placed directly over a wound to help absorb blood, prevent infection, and protect the wound from further injury. Dressings come in different shapes, sizes, and types. Dressings can be gauze pads (for example, 10 cm square or larger) used to cover larger wounds, or adhesive strips such as Band-Aids, which are dressings combined with a bandage for small cuts or scrapes **Figure 5-4**. It is often preferable to use non-adhesive, absorbent (NAA) dressings to wounds, as this ensures that fluff does not become attached to the wound and also the dressing can be lifted without adhering to the wound to allow further inspection if necessary.

A **bandage**, such as a roll of gauze, is often used to cover a dressing to keep it in place on the wound and to apply pressure to help control the bleeding. Like dressings, bandages also come in different shapes, sizes, and material **Figure 5-5**. Elastic bandages can be used to provide support and stability for an extremity or joint and to reduce swelling. In most first aid at work kits, dressings come readily attached to bandages.

When commercial bandages are unavailable, you can improvise bandages from ties, handkerchiefs, or strips of cloth torn from a sheet or other similar material.

When applying a bandage, do not apply it so tightly that it restricts blood circulation. The signs that a bandage is too tight are as follows:

- Blue tinge to the fingernails or toenails
- Blue or pale skin
- Tingling or loss of sensation
- Coldness of the extremity

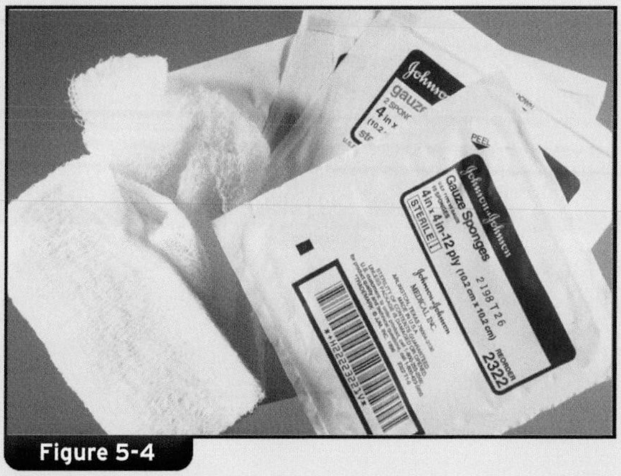

Figure 5-4

Dressings.

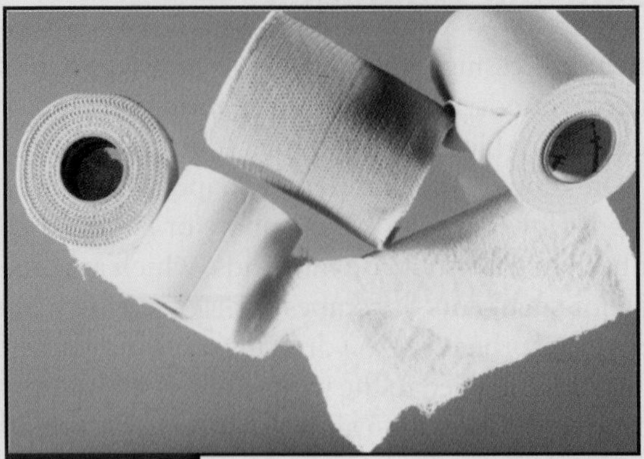

Figure 5-5

Bandages.

First Aid Objectives

This chapter covers the following guidelines for First Aid training and will enable the student to be able to:

- Act safely, promptly, and effectively with emergencies at work.
- Use First Aid equipment, including the contents of the First Aid box.
- Recognise the importance of personal hygiene in First Aid procedures.
- Deal with a casualty who is bleeding or wounded.

Bleeding

What to Look For	What to Do
External Bleeding • Blood coming from an open wound	1. Protect against blood contact. 2. Place sterile dressing over wound and apply pressure. 3. Elevate the injured area if possible. 4. Apply a pressure bandage. 5. If bleeding cannot be controlled, apply pressure to a pressure point. 6. Apply a tourniquet to the affected limb if all other methods fail.
Internal Bleeding • Bruising • Painful, tender area • Vomiting or coughing up blood • Stool that is black or contains bright red blood	Minor internal bleeding: 1. Use RICE procedures: • R = Rest • I = Ice or cold pack • C = Compress the area with elastic bandage • E = Elevate the injured extremity Serious internal bleeding: 1. Call 9-9-9 or 1-1-2. 2. Care for shock. 3. If vomiting occurs, roll the casualty onto side.

Wounds

What to Look For	What to Do
Wound Care	1. Wash with soap and water. 2. Flush with running water under pressure. 3. Remove remaining small object(s). 4. If the bleeding restarts, apply pressure on wound. 5. Cover with sterile or clean dressing. 6. For wounds with a high risk for infection, seek medical care for cleaning, possible tetanus booster, and closing.
Amputation • Loss of a body part	1. Call 9-9-9 or 1-1-2. 2. Control bleeding. 3. Care for shock. 4. Recover amputated part(s) and wrap in clean plastic or cling film. 5. Place wrapped part(s) in a clean dressing or cloth. 6. Keep part(s) cool.

prep kit

▶ Key Terms

<u>arterial bleeding</u> Bleeding from an artery; this type of bleeding tends to spurt with each heartbeat.

<u>bandage</u> Used to cover a dressing to keep it in place on the wound and to apply pressure to help control bleeding.

<u>capillary bleeding</u> Bleeding that oozes from a wound steadily but slowly.

<u>dressing</u> A sterile gauze pad or clean cloth covering placed over an open wound.

<u>haemorrhage</u> A large amount of bleeding in a short time.

<u>venous bleeding</u> Bleeding from a vein; this type of bleeding tends to flow steadily.

▶ Assessment in Action

A 25-year-old carpenter has been badly cut on his thigh by a circular power saw. The cut is approximately 15 cm long, and blood is spurting from the wound.

Directions: Circle Yes if you agree with the statement, and circle No if you disagree.

Yes No **1.** This casualty is experiencing venous bleeding.

Yes No **2.** You should be certain to wash this wound with soap and water.

Yes No **3.** Direct pressure should stop the bleeding.

Yes No **4.** Treat the casualty for shock.

Yes No **5.** The type of bleeding experienced by this man is the most common type.

Answers: **1.** No; **2.** No; **3.** Yes; **4.** Yes; **5.** No

▶ Check Your Knowledge

Directions: Circle Yes if you agree with the statement, and circle No if you disagree.

Yes No **1.** Most cases of bleeding require more than direct pressure to stop the bleeding.

Yes No **2.** Remove any blood-soaked dressings before applying additional ones.

Yes No **3.** Whenever elevating an arm or leg to control bleeding, you should also keep applying pressure on the wound.

Yes No **4.** If a bleeding arm wound is not controlled through direct pressure, elevation, and pressure bandaging, apply pressure to the brachial artery.

Yes No **5.** Dressings are placed directly on a wound.

Yes No **6.** Care for an amputated part by placing it in a container of water to keep it moist and clean.

Yes No **7.** Dressings should be sterile or as clean as possible.

Yes No **8.** Antibiotic ointments can be placed on any open wound.

Yes No **9.** Keep an amputated part packed in ice to preserve it.

Answers: **1.** No; **2.** No; **3.** Yes; **4.** Yes; **5.** Yes; **6.** No; **7.** Yes; **8.** No; **9.** No

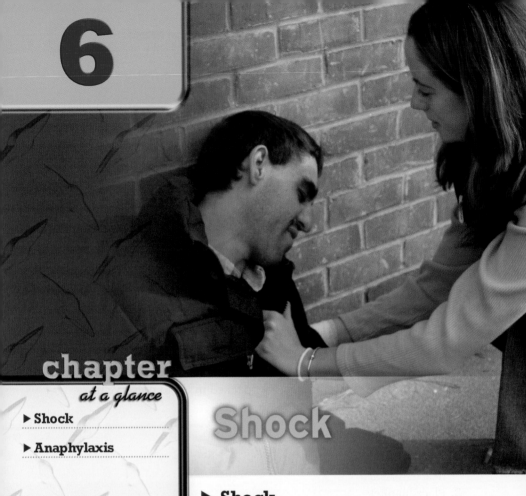

6

chapter *at a glance*

▸ Shock

▸ Anaphylaxis

Shock

▸ Shock

Shock occurs when the body's tissues do not receive enough oxygenated blood. Do not confuse this with an electric shock or "being shocked," as in being scared or surprised. To understand shock, think of the circulatory system as having three components: a working pump (the heart), a network of pipes (the blood vessels), and an adequate amount of fluid (the blood) pumped through the pipes. Damage to any of the components can deprive tissues of oxygen-rich blood and produce the condition known as shock.

Recognising Shock

The signs of shock include the following:

- Altered mental status:
  - Agitation
  - Anxiety
  - Restlessness
  - Confusion
- Pale, cold, and clammy skin, lips, and nail beds
- Nausea and vomiting
- Rapid breathing
- Unresponsiveness (when shock is severe)
- As a casualty deteriorates, their breathing and pulse rate will increase whilst their level of consciousness will decrease. It is important to regularly assess these vital signs to recognise whether your casualty's condition is becoming worse.

Care for Shock

Even if there are no signs of shock, you should still treat seriously injured and suddenly ill casualties for shock.

1. Place the casualty on his or her back.
2. Raise the legs approximately 30 cm (if spinal injury is not suspected). Raising the legs allows the blood to drain from the legs back to the heart **Figure 6-1**.
3. Place blankets under and over the casualty to keep the casualty warm.

Other positions may be used in shock when other conditions are present **Figure 6-2 A-D**.

▶ Anaphylaxis

A life-threatening breathing emergency can result from a severe allergic reaction called anaphylaxis. This reaction happens when a substance to which the casualty is very sensitive enters the body. It can be deadly within minutes if untreated. Many of the deaths are caused by the inability to breathe because swollen airway passages block air to the lungs. The most common causes of anaphylaxis include the following:

- Medications (for example, penicillin and related drugs, aspirin)
- Food (for example, nuts, especially peanuts; eggs; shellfish)
- Insect stings (for example, honeybee, wasp, hornet)
- Plants (for example, inhaled pollen)

Figure 6-1

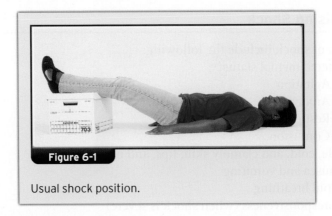

Usual shock position.

Recognising Anaphylaxis

The most common signs of anaphylaxis include the following:

- Breathing difficulty—shortness of breath and wheezing
- Skin reaction—itching or burning skin, especially over the face and upper part of the chest, with rash or hives
- Swelling of the lips, mouth, tongue, or throat, or around the eyes

Other signs of anaphylaxis are as follows:

- Sneezing, coughing
- Tightness in the chest
- Blueness around lips and mouth
- Dizziness
- Nausea and vomiting

Care for Anaphylaxis

To care for anaphylaxis:

1. Call 9-9-9 or 1-1-2.
2. Determine whether the casualty has medication for allergic reactions. If the casualty has a prescribed adrenaline auto-injector, help the casualty use it. If you are assisting with or using an auto-injector, follow these steps:
   - Remove the safety cap. The auto-injector is now ready for use.
   - Support the casualty's thigh and place the black tip of the auto-injector lightly against the outer thigh.
   - Using a quick motion, push the auto-injector firmly against the thigh and hold it in place for several seconds. This will inject the medication.
   - Remove the auto-injector from the thigh. Carefully reinsert the used auto-injector, needle first, into the carrying tube. A small amount of medication will remain in the device, but the device cannot be reused.
3. Keep a responsive casualty sitting up to help breathing. Place an unresponsive casualty in the recovery position.

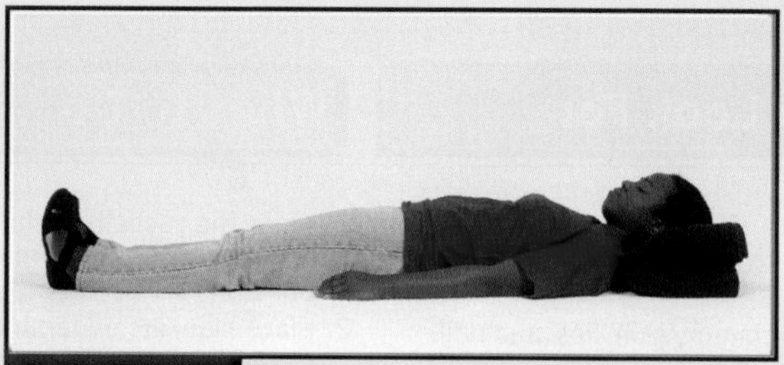

Figure 6-2A

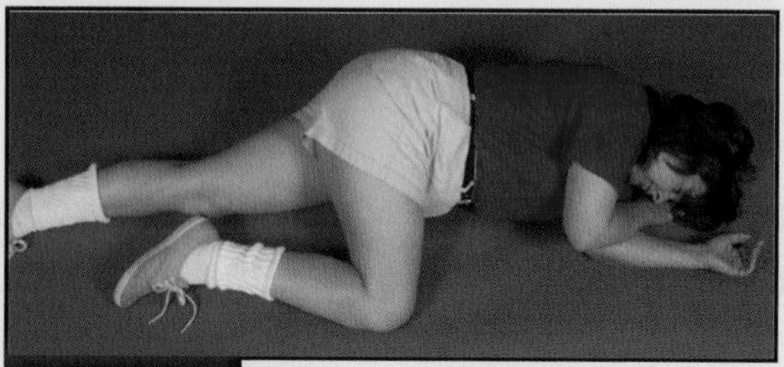

Figure 6-2B

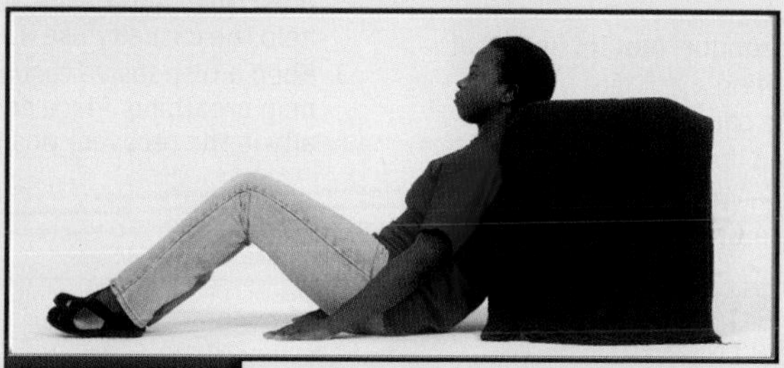

Figure 6-2C

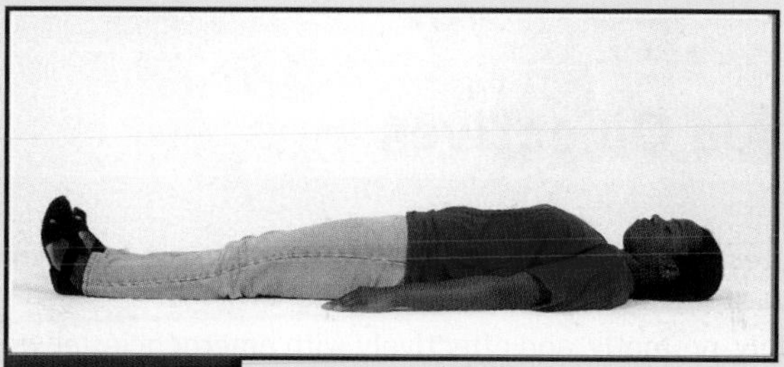

Figure 6-2D

Other positions that may be used in certain cases of shock. **A.** For a casualty with head injury, elevate the head (if spinal injury is not suspected). **B.** Position an unresponsive or stroke casualty in the recovery position. **C.** Use a half-sitting position for casualties with breathing difficulties, chest injuries, or a heart attack. **D.** Keep the casualty flat if a spinal injury or leg fracture is suspected.

Shock

What to Look For

Shock
- Altered mental status (anxiety, restlessness)
- Pale, cold, and clammy skin, lips, and nail beds
- Nausea and vomiting
- Rapid breathing

What to Do

1. Place the casualty on his or her back and raise the legs approximately 30 cm. Other positions are used for other conditions.
2. Place blankets under and over the casualty to keep the casualty warm.

Anaphylaxis

What to Look For

Anaphylaxis
- Breathing difficulty
- Skin reaction
- Swelling of the tongue, mouth, or throat
- Sneezing, coughing
- Tightness in the chest
- Blueness around lips and mouth
- Dizziness
- Nausea and vomiting

What to Do

1. Call 9-9-9 or 1-1-2.
2. Determine whether casualty has a prescribed adrenaline auto-injector and help the casualty use it.
3. Keep a responsive casualty sitting up to help breathing. Place an unresponsive casualty in the recovery position.

First Aid Objectives

This chapter covers the following guidelines for First Aid training and will enable the student to be able to:

- Act safely, promptly, and effectively with emergencies at work.
- Deal with a casualty who is suffering from shock.

prep kit

▶ Key Terms

adrenaline auto-injector Prescribed device used to administer an emergency dose of adrenaline to a casualty experiencing anaphylaxis.

anaphylaxis A life-threatening allergic reaction.

shock Inadequate tissue oxygenation resulting from serious injury or illness.

▶ Assessment in Action

A woman was working in her garden on a warm summer day. She unintentionally disturbed a nest of wasps and was stung several times on her face and neck. She has begun coughing and wheezing. She complains that she is dizzy and having difficulty breathing. You notice that her face is swelling.

Directions: Circle Yes if you agree with the statement, and circle No if you disagree.

Yes No 1. Breathing difficulty and swelling may be signs of a severe allergic reaction.

Yes No 2. This casualty is likely experiencing a type of shock known as anaphylaxis.

Yes No 3. The condition this casualty is experiencing is life threatening, and medical care is needed.

Yes No 4. If the casualty has a prescribed adrenaline auto-injector, help her use it.

Yes No 5. Place this casualty in the usual shock position—lying down with the legs raised.

Answers: **1.** Yes; **2.** Yes; **3.** Yes; **4.** Yes; **5.** No

▶ Check Your Knowledge

Directions: Circle Yes if you agree with the statement, and circle No if you disagree.

Yes No 1. Raise the legs of all severely injured casualties.

Yes No 2. Prevent body heat loss by putting blankets under and over the casualty.

Yes No 3. A shock casualty with possible spinal injuries should be placed in a seated position.

Yes No 4. A shock casualty with breathing difficulty or chest injury should be placed on his or her back with the legs raised.

Yes No 5. Anxiety and restlessness are signs of shock.

Yes No 6. An adrenaline auto-injector requires a doctor's prescription.

Yes No 7. All severely injured or ill casualties should be treated for shock.

Yes No 8. Treat severely injured casualties for shock even though there are no signs of it.

Yes No 9. Anaphylaxis is a life-threatening breathing emergency.

Yes No 10. Casualties in shock have hot skin.

Answers: **1.** No; **2.** Yes; **3.** No; **4.** No; **5.** Yes; **6.** Yes; **7.** Yes; **8.** Yes; **9.** Yes; **10.** No

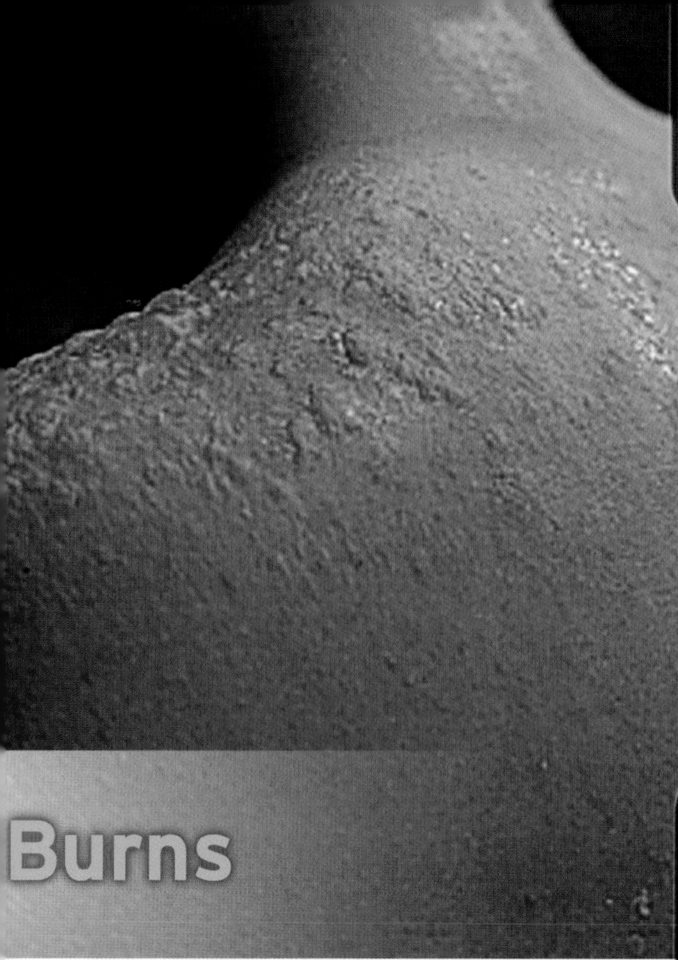

chapter 7

Burns

chapter *at a glance*

- Types of Burns
- Thermal Burns
- Care for Thermal Burns
- Chemical Burns
- Electrical Burns

Types of Burns

Burn injuries can be classified as thermal (heat), chemical, or electrical.

▶ Thermal Burns

Thermal (heat) burns can be caused by flames, contact with hot objects, steam, or hot liquid.

Superficial burns affect the skin's outer layer (epidermis) **Figure 7-1**. Characteristics include redness, mild swelling, tenderness, and pain. Sunburn is a common example of a superficial burn.

Partial-thickness burns extend through the skin's entire outer layer and into the inner layer **Figure 7-2**. Blisters, swelling, weeping of fluids, and pain identify these burns.

Full-thickness burns are severe burns that penetrate all of the skin layers and the underlying fat and muscle. The skin looks leathery, waxy, or pearly grey, and sometimes charred. The casualty feels no pain from a full-thickness burn because the nerve endings have been damaged or destroyed.

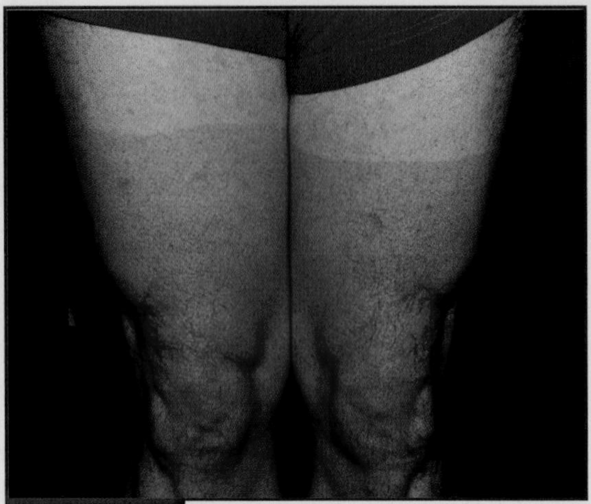

Figure 7-1

Superficial burn.

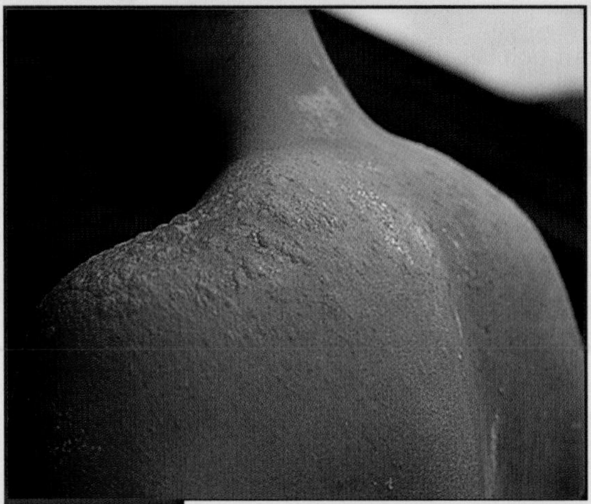

Figure 7-2

Partial-thickness burn.

▶ Care for Thermal Burns

Burn care aims to reduce pain and protect against infection.

Care for Superficial Burns

1. Cool the burn with cold water until the part is pain free (at least 10 minutes) Figure 7-3.
2. Put on gloves.
3. Remove any constrictive jewellery or clothing prior to the area swelling.

Care for Small Partial-Thickness Burns

1. Cool the burn with cold water until the part is pain free (at least 10 minutes).
2. Put on gloves.
3. Cover the burn loosely with a dry, non-adhesive, sterile or clean dressing to keep the burn clean, prevent evaporative moisture loss, and reduce pain.

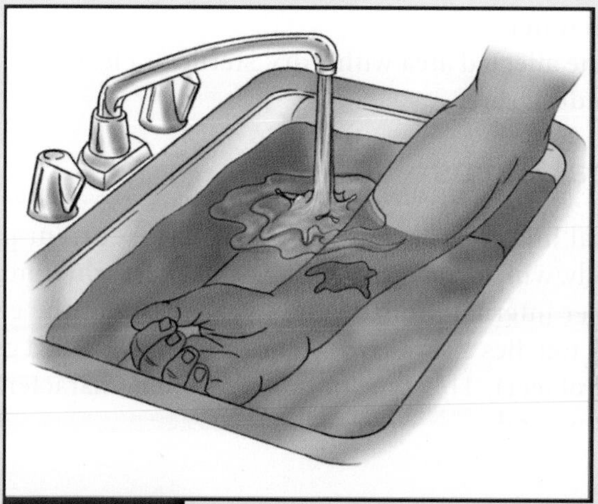

Figure 7-3

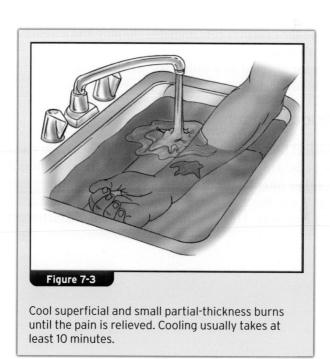

Cool superficial and small partial-thickness burns until the pain is relieved. Cooling usually takes at least 10 minutes.

Care for Large Partial-Thickness and Full-Thickness Burns

1. Call 9-9-9 or 1-1-2.
2. Remove clothing and jewellery that is not stuck to the burned area.
3. Put on gloves.
4. Cover the burn with a dry, non-adhesive, sterile or clean dressing. If dressings are not available, consider food standard grade cling film. This should be applied in long strips and must not be wrapped around a limb, as this would cause a tourniquet effect if swelling occurs.
5. Monitor the casualty.

▶ Chemical Burns

A chemical burn results when a caustic or corrosive substance touches the skin. Examples of such substances include acids, alkalis, and organic compounds. Because chemicals continue to burn as long as they are in contact with the skin, they should be removed from the skin as rapidly as possible.

Care for Chemical Burns

1. Put on gloves.
2. Immediately flush the area with a large quantity of water for 20 minutes. If the chemical is a dry powder, brush the powder from the skin before flushing.
3. Remove the casualty's contaminated clothing and jewellery while flushing with water.
4. Cover the affected area with a dry, sterile or clean dressing.
5. Seek medical care.

▶ Electrical Burns

A true electrical injury happens when an electric current passes directly through the body, which can disrupt the normal heart rhythm and cause cardiac arrest, other internal injuries, and burns. Usually, the electricity exits where the body touches a surface or comes in contact with a ground (for example, a metal object). This type of injury is often characterised by an entrance and exit wound.

Care for Electrical Burns

1. Make sure the area is safe. Unplug, disconnect, or turn off the power. If that is impossible, call 9-9-9 or 1-1-2.
2. Monitor breathing.
3. If the casualty fell, check for a possible spinal injury.
4. Care for shock.
5. Call 9-9-9 or 1-1-2 for medical care.

First Aid Objectives

This chapter covers the following guidelines for First Aid training and will enable the student to be able to:

- Act safely, promptly, and effectively with emergencies at work.
- Use First Aid equipment.
- Deal with a casualty who has been burned or scalded.

Thermal (Heat) Burns

What to Look For

Superficial Burn
- Redness
- Mild swelling
- Pain

What to Do

1. Cool the burn with cold water.
2. Seek advice for pain relief.

What to Look For

Partial-Thickness Burn
- Blisters
- Swelling
- Pain
- Weeping of fluid

What to Do

1. Cool the burn with cold water.
2. Cover with a dry, non-adhesive, sterile dressing.
3. If no dressings are available, consider using food grade cling film, applied lengthways to limb.
4. Seek medical care.

What to Look For

Full-Thickness Burn
- Dry, leathery skin
- Grey or charred skin

What to Do

1. Seek medical care.
2. Monitor breathing and provide care as needed.
3. Cover burn with a dry, non-adhesive, sterile or clean dressing.
4. Care for shock.

Chemical Burns

What to Look For

Chemical Burn
- Stinging pain

What to Do

1. Brush dry powder chemicals off skin.
2. Flush with a large amount of water for 20 minutes.
3. Remove casualty's contaminated clothing and jewellery while flushing.
4. Cover area with a dry, sterile or clean dressing.
5. Seek medical care.

Electrical Burns

What to Look For

Electrical Burn
- Possible full-thickness burn with entrance and exit wounds

What to Do

1. Safety first! Unplug, disconnect, or turn off the electricity.
2. Open the airway, check breathing, and provide care as needed.
3. Care for electrical burns as you would a full-thickness burn.
4. Call 9-9-9 or 1-1-2.

prep kit

▶ Key Terms

full-thickness burn A burn that penetrates all the skin layers into the underlying fat and muscle.

partial-thickness burn A burn that extends through the skin's entire outer layer and into the inner layer.

superficial burn A burn that affects the skin's outer layer.

▶ Assessment in Action

At a fast-food restaurant, a worker is burned on his forearm after bumping into a hot pan on the stove. The burned area is about the width of a tennis ball. Blisters are forming and the worker complains about the pain.

Directions: Circle Yes if you agree with the statement, and circle No if you disagree.

Yes No **1.** The blisters and pain are signs that the burn is a full-thickness burn.

Yes No **2.** Reduce the pain and damage by running cold water over the burned area.

Yes No **3.** An antibiotic ointment can be applied to this burn only after cooling the area.

Yes No **4.** This casualty needs medical care.

Answers: **1.** No; **2.** Yes; **3.** No; **4.** No

▶ Check Your Knowledge

Directions: Circle Yes if you agree with the statement, and circle No if you disagree.

Yes No **1.** The hands and feet are especially sensitive to being burned.

Yes No **2.** Petroleum jelly can be applied over a burn.

Yes No **3.** Use a large amount of water to flush chemicals off the body.

Yes No **4.** Brush a dry chemical off the skin before flushing with water.

Yes No **5.** When someone gets electrocuted, there can be two burn wounds: entrance and exit.

Yes No **6.** When a casualty is in contact with a power line, use a tree branch to remove the wires.

Yes No **7.** Seek medical advice before giving pain relief.

Yes No **8.** Cold water can be used on any burn of any size.

Answers: **1.** Yes; **2.** No; **3.** Yes; **4.** Yes; **5.** Yes; **6.** No; **7.** Yes; **8.** No

8

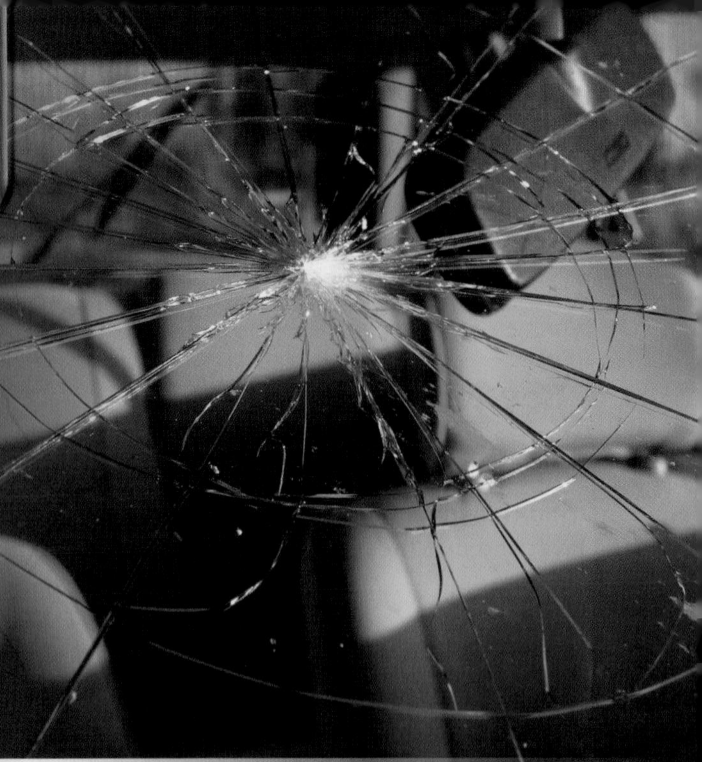

chapter
at a glance

- Head Injuries
- Eye Injuries
- Nose Injuries
- Spinal Injuries

Head and Spinal Injuries

Head Injuries

Any head injury is potentially serious. If not properly treated, injuries that seem minor could become life threatening. Head injuries include scalp wounds, skull fractures, and brain injuries. Spinal injuries (that is, neck and back injuries) can also be present in head-injured casualties.

▶ Scalp Wounds

The scalp has many blood vessels, so any cut can cause heavy bleeding. A bleeding scalp wound does not affect the blood supply to the brain.

Care for Scalp Wounds

To care for a scalp wound:

1. Apply a sterile or clean dressing and direct pressure to control bleeding Figure 8-1.
2. Keep the casualty's head and shoulders slightly elevated to help control bleeding if no spinal injury is suspected.
3. Seek medical care.

CAUTION

DO NOT remove an embedded object; instead, stabilise it in place with bulky dressings.

DO NOT clean or irrigate a scalp wound if you suspect a skull fracture, because the fluid can carry debris and bacteria into the brain.

▶ Skull Fracture

Significant force applied to the head may cause a skull fracture. This occurs when part of the skull (the bones forming the head) is broken.

Recognising Skull Fracture

Signs of skull fracture include the following:

- Pain at the point of injury
- Deformity of the skull
- Drainage of clear or bloody fluid from the ears or nose

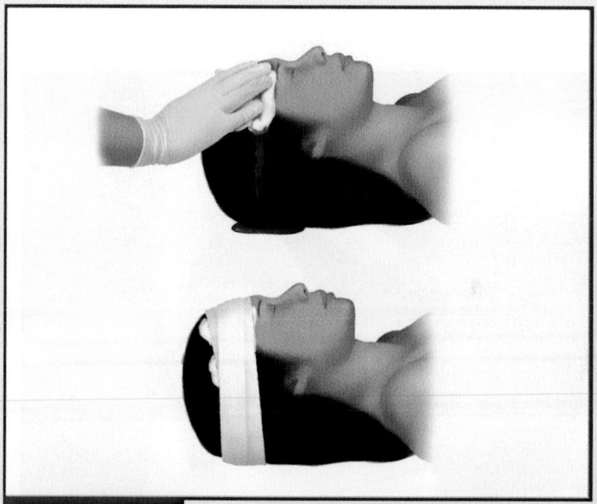

Figure 8-1

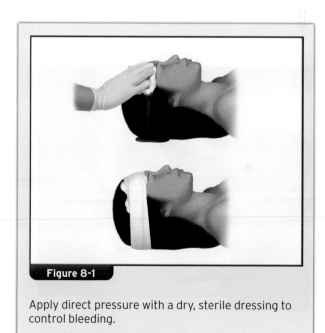

Apply direct pressure with a dry, sterile dressing to control bleeding.

- Bruising under the eyes or behind an ear appearing several hours after the injury
- Changes in pupils (unequal, not reactive to light)
- Heavy scalp bleeding (a scalp wound may expose the skull or brain tissue)
- Penetrating wound, such as from a bullet or an impaled object

Care for Skull Fracture

To care for a skull fracture:

1. Monitor breathing and provide care if needed.
2. Control any bleeding by applying a sterile or clean dressing and applying pressure around the edges of the wound, not directly on it Figure 8-2.
3. Stabilise the head and neck to prevent movement.
4. Seek medical care.

▶ Brain Injuries

The brain can be shaken by a blow to the head. A temporary disturbance of brain activity known as a concussion can result. Most concussions are mild, and people recover fully, but this process takes time. A more serious brain injury occurs when bleeding between the skull and the brain causes a build up of pressure, often referred to as cerebral compression. This pressure, or bleed, pushes on the brain and may eventually cause the casualty to become unconscious. In some situations, the pressure may build up over a period of days.

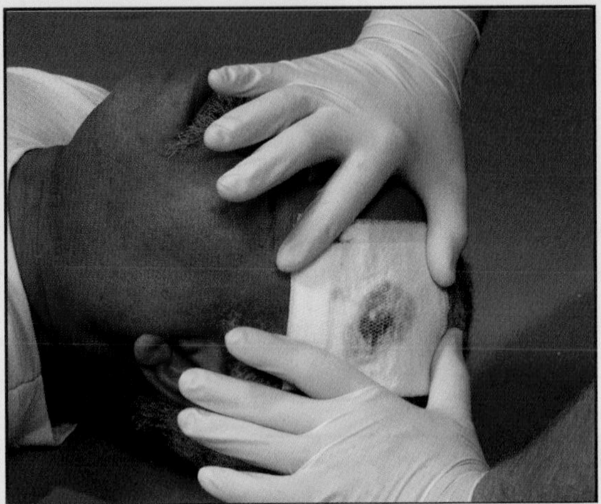

Figure 8-2

Apply pressure around the edges of the wound to control bleeding from a suspected skull fracture.

Recognising Brain Injury

Signs of brain injury include the following:

- Befuddled facial expression (vacant stare)
- Unawareness of where they are or what day of the week it is
- Slowness in answering questions
- Slurred speech
- Headache and dizziness
- Nausea and vomiting
- Visual problems, unequal pupils
- Stumbling, inability to walk a straight line
- Weakness or paralysis to limbs
- Drowsiness, mood change
- Unconsciousness

Care for Brain Injuries

To care for a brain injury:

1. Monitor breathing and provide care if needed.
2. Stabilise the head and neck to prevent movement.
3. Control any scalp bleeding with a sterile or clean dressing and direct pressure. If you suspect a skull fracture, apply pressure around the wound edges, not directly on the wound.
4. If the casualty vomits, roll the casualty onto his or her side to keep the airway clear, moving the head, neck, and body as one unit.
5. Seek medical care.

CAUTION

DO NOT stop the flow of fluid from the ears or nose. Blocking the flow of either could increase pressure inside the skull.

DO NOT elevate the legs—that might increase pressure on the brain.

DO NOT clean an open skull injury—infection of the brain may result.

Eye Injuries

Eye injuries are common, particularly in sports. An eye injury can produce severe lifelong complications, including blindness. When in doubt about an injury's severity, seek medical care.

▶ Foreign Objects in Eye

Many different types of objects can enter the eye and cause significant damage. Even a small foreign object, such as a grain of sand, can produce severe irritation.

Care for Loose Foreign Objects in Eye

Try one or more of the following techniques to remove the object Figure 8-3.

1. Lift the upper lid over the lower lid, so that the lower lashes can brush the object off the inside of the upper lid. Have the casualty blink a few times.
2. Hold the eyelid open, and gently rinse with running water or use pre-bottled eyewash liquid.
3. Examine the lower lid by pulling it down gently. If you can see the object, remove it with moistened sterile gauze or a clean cloth.
4. Examine the underside of the upper lid by grasping the lashes of the upper lid and rolling the lid upward over a stick or swab. If you can see the object, remove it with moistened sterile gauze or a clean cloth.

CAUTION

DO NOT allow the casualty to rub the eye.

DO NOT try to remove an embedded foreign object.

DO NOT use dry cotton (cotton balls or cotton-tipped swabs) or instruments such as tweezers to remove an object from an eye.

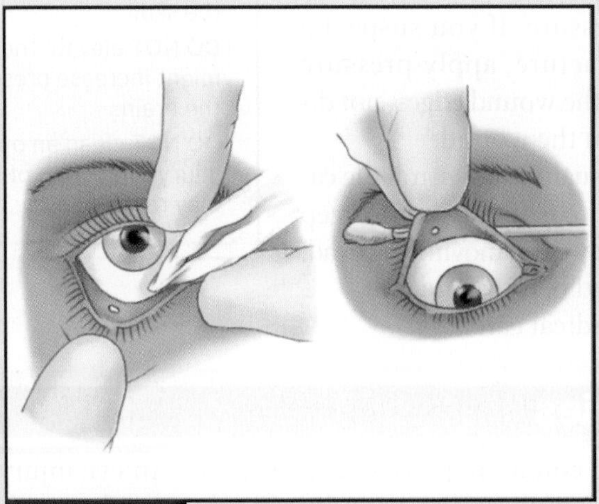

Figure 8-3

Locate and remove a foreign object from the eye.

▶ Chemicals in the Eye

Chemical burns of the eye, usually caused by an acid or alkaline solution, need immediate care because damage can occur in as little as 1 minute. They may cause the loss of vision.

Care for Chemicals in the Eye

To care for a chemical in the eye:

1. Hold the eye wide open and flush with running water or pre-bottled eyewash liquid for at least 20 minutes, continuously and gently (Figure 8-4). Irrigate from the nose side of the eye toward the outside to avoid flushing material into the other eye.
2. Loosely bandage the eyes with wet dressings.
3. Seek medical care.

CAUTION

DO NOT try to neutralise the chemical. Water is usually readily available and is better for eye irrigation.

DO NOT bandage the eye tightly.

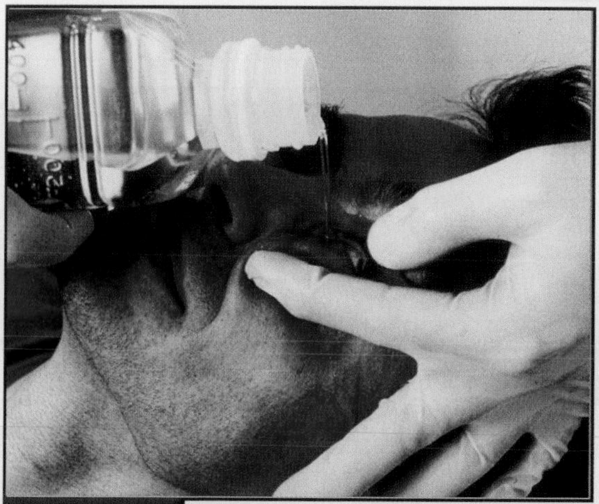

Figure 8-4

Flushing eye to treat a chemical burn.

Nose Injuries

The nose often gets hit during sports activities, physical assaults, and road traffic collisions.

▶ Nosebleeds

Rupture of tiny blood vessels inside the nostrils by a blow to the nose, sneezing, or picking or blowing the nose causes most nosebleeds.

There are two types of nosebleeds:

- Anterior nosebleeds (front of nose) are the most common type of nosebleed (90%) and are normally easily cared for.
- A posterior nosebleed (back of nose) involves massive bleeding backward into the mouth or down the back of the throat. A posterior nosebleed is serious and requires medical care.

Care for Nosebleeds

To care for a nosebleed:

1. Place the casualty in a seated position with the casualty's head tilted slightly forward.
2. Pinch (or have the casualty pinch) the soft parts of the nose between the thumb and two fingers with steady pressure for 5 to 10 minutes Figure 8-5.

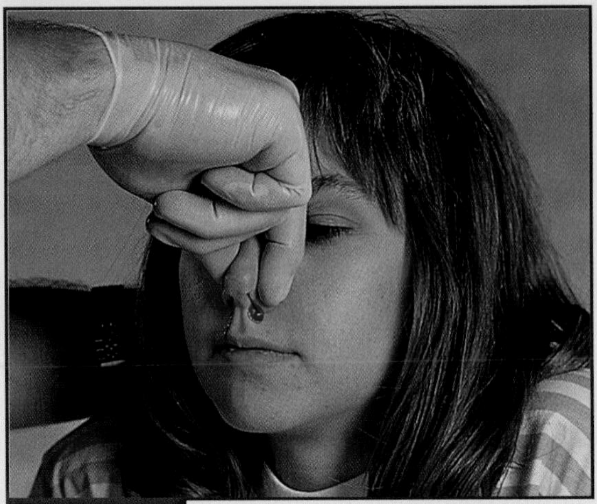

Figure 8-5

Control bleeding from the nose by pinching the nostrils together.

3. Seek medical care if any of the following applies:
   - Bleeding cannot be controlled.
   - You suspect a posterior nosebleed.
   - The casualty has high blood pressure or is taking anticoagulants (blood thinners) or large doses of aspirin.
   - Bleeding occurs after a blow to the nose, and you suspect a broken nose.

CAUTION

DO NOT allow the casualty to tilt his or her head backward.

DO NOT probe the nose with a cotton-tipped swab.

DO NOT move the casualty's head and neck if a spinal injury is suspected.

▶ Broken Nose

A blow to the nose can break the nose.

Recognising a Broken Nose

The signs of a broken nose include the following:

- Pain, swelling, and possibly crooked nose
- Bleeding and breathing difficulty through the nostrils
- Black eyes appearing 1 to 2 days after the injury

Care for a Broken Nose

To care for a broken nose:

1. If bleeding, provide care as for a nosebleed.
2. Apply an ice or cold pack to the nose for 10 minutes. Do not try to straighten a crooked nose.
3. Seek medical care.

Spinal Injuries

Road traffic collisions, direct blows, falls from heights, physical assaults, and sports injuries are common causes of spinal injury. Suspect spine injuries in casualties with significant head injuries, since the two are often associated.

Recognising Spinal Injuries

The signs of spinal injuries include the following:

- Inability to move arms and/or legs
- Numbness, tingling, weakness, or burning sensation in the arms and/or legs
- Deformity (odd-looking angle of the casualty's head and neck)
- Neck or back pain

Care for Spinal Injuries

To care for a spinal injury:

1. Stabilise the head and neck to prevent movement Figure 8-6.
2. If unresponsive, open the airway, check breathing, and provide any needed care.
3. Call 9-9-9 or 1-1-2.

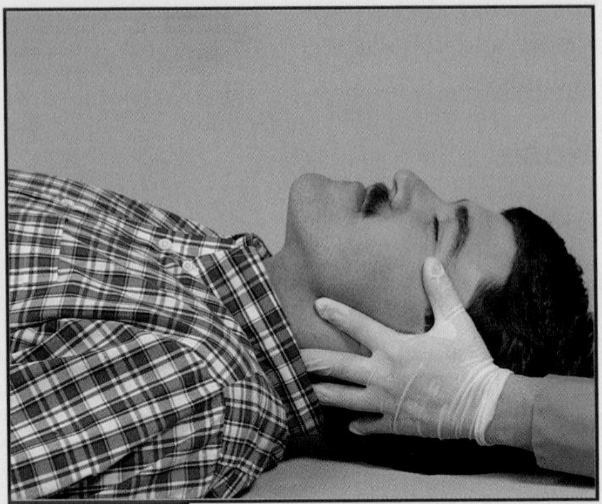

Figure 8-6

Prevent movement of the head and neck.

First Aid Objectives

This chapter covers the following guidelines for First Aid training and will enable the student to be able to:

- Act safely, promptly, and effectively with emergencies at work.
- Use First Aid equipment, including the contents of a First Aid box.
- Recognise the importance of personal hygiene in First Aid procedures.

Head Injuries

What to Look For	What to Do
Scalp Wound	1. Apply a sterile or clean dressing and direct pressure to control bleeding. 2. Keep head and shoulders raised. 3. Seek medical care.
Skull Fracture • Pain at point of injury • Deformity of the skull • Clear or bloody fluid draining from ears or nose • Bruising under eyes or behind an ear • Changes in pupils • Heavy scalp bleeding • Penetrating wound	1. Monitor breathing and provide care if needed. 2. Control bleeding by applying pressure around the edges of wound. 3. Stabilise the casualty's head and neck against movement. 4. Seek medical care.
Brain Injury (Concussion) • Befuddled facial expression (vacant stare) • Slowness in answering questions • Unawareness of where they are or day of week • Slurred speech • Stumbling, inability to walk a straight line • Crying for no apparent reason • Inability to recite months of year in reverse order • Unresponsiveness • Headache, dizziness, and nausea	1. Monitor breathing and provide care if needed. 2. Stabilise the casualty's head and neck against movement. 3. Control any scalp bleeding. 4. Seek medical care.

Eye Injuries

What to Look For	What to Do
Loose Foreign Object in Eye	1. Look for object underneath both lids. 2. If seen, remove with wet gauze.
Chemicals in Eye	1. Flush with water for 20 minutes and loosely bandage with wet dressings. 2. Seek medical care.

Nose Injuries

What to Look For	What to Do
Nosebleeds	1. Keep casualty sitting up with head level or tilted forward slightly. 2. Pinch soft parts of nose for 5 to 10 minutes. 3. Seek medical care if: • Bleeding does not stop • Blood is going down throat • Bleeding is associated with a broken nose
Broken Nose • Pain, swelling, and possibly crooked nose • Bleeding and breathing difficulty through nostrils • Black eyes appearing 1 to 2 days after injury	1. Care for nosebleed. 2. Apply an ice or cold pack for 10 minutes. 3. Seek medical care.

Spinal Injuries

What to Look For	What to Do
Spinal Injury • Inability to move arms and/or legs • Numbness, tingling, weakness, or burning feeling in arms and/or legs • Deformity (head and neck at an odd angle) • Neck or back pain	1. Stabilise the head and neck against movement. 2. If unresponsive, open the casualty's airway and check breathing. 3. Call 9-9-9 or 1-1-2.

prep kit

▶ Key Terms

anterior nosebleed Bleeding from the front of the nose.

concussion A temporary disturbance of brain activity caused by a blow to the head.

posterior nosebleed Bleeding from the back of the nose into the mouth or down the back of the throat.

skull fracture A break of part of the skull (head bones).

▶ Assessment in Action

You see a middle-aged man walking down the street; suddenly, he is struck by a piece of wood that has fallen 20 metres from a building site above. The casualty collapses and remains on the ground. He is slow to answer questions and cannot remember where he is or the day of the week. He says he feels lightheaded and nauseated. You see a lot of blood coming from a wound on his head.

Directions: Circle Yes if you agree with the statement, and circle No if you disagree.

Yes No **1.** Head-injured casualties should be checked for possible spinal injury.

Yes No **2.** You think the casualty may have suffered a skull fracture, so you press around the wound's edges rather than applying hard pressure over the wound to control the bleeding.

Yes No **3.** To treat for shock, this casualty should be placed flat on his back with his legs elevated.

Yes No **4.** You do not suspect a concussion because the casualty is still alert.

Yes No **5.** Minimise head and neck movement by not touching the casualty—leave him as you found him.

Answers: **1.** Yes; **2.** Yes; **3.** No; **4.** No; **5.** Yes

▶ Check Your Knowledge

Directions: Circle Yes if you agree with the statement, and circle No if you disagree.

Yes No **1.** Scalp wounds have very little bleeding.

Yes No **2.** Tears are sufficient to flush a chemical from the eye.

Yes No **3.** Use clean, damp gauze to remove an object from the eyelid's surface.

Yes No **4.** Do not move a casualty with a suspected spinal injury.

Yes No **5.** Inability to move the hands or feet, or both, may indicate a spinal injury.

Yes No **6.** To care for a nosebleed, have the injured person sit down and tilt his or her head back.

Answers: **1.** No; **2.** No; **3.** Yes; **4.** Yes; **5.** Yes; **6.** No

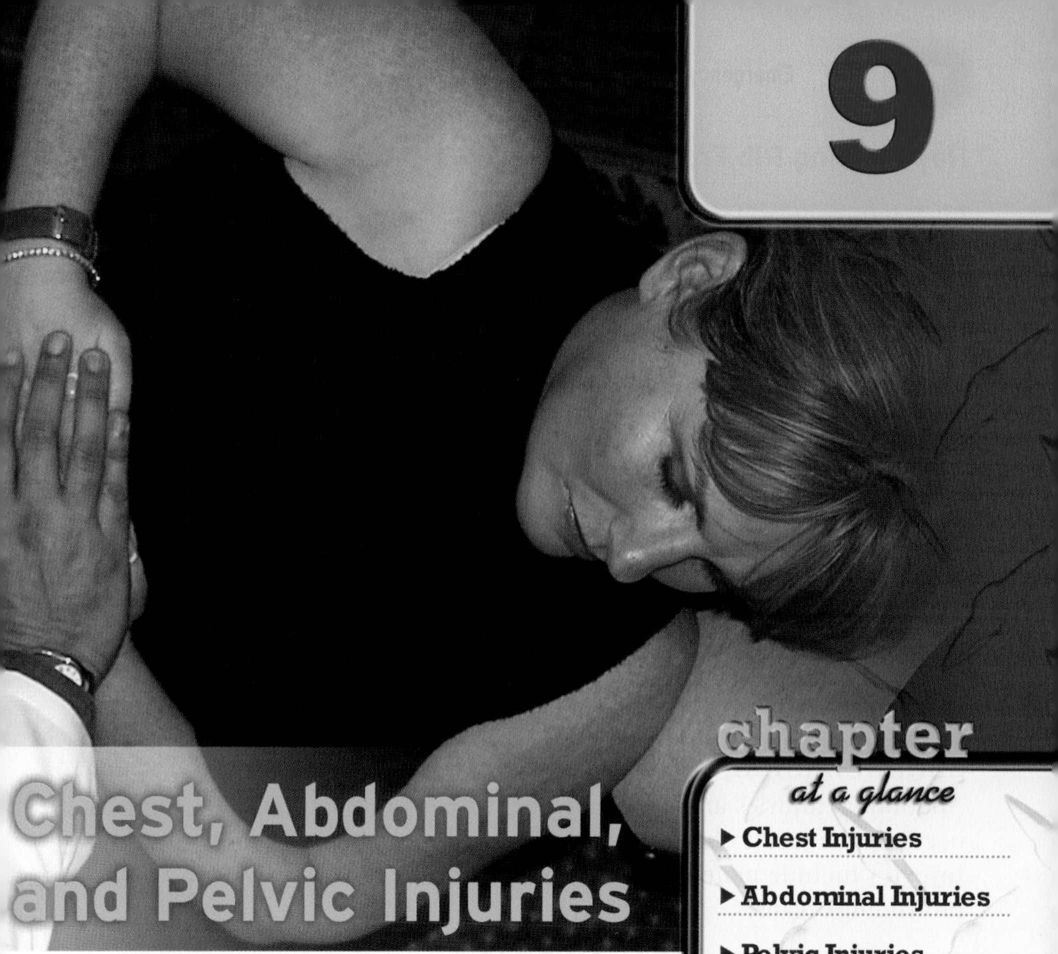

9

Chest, Abdominal, and Pelvic Injuries

chapter *at a glance*

- Chest Injuries
- Abdominal Injuries
- Pelvic Injuries

▶ Chest Injuries

Chest injuries can be closed or open. In a closed chest injury, the casualty's skin is not broken. This type of injury is usually caused by blunt trauma. In an open chest injury, the skin has been broken and the chest wall is penetrated by an object such as a knife, bullet, or piece of machinery.

A responsive chest injury casualty should usually sit up or, if the injury is on a side, be placed with the injured side down. This position prevents blood inside the chest cavity from seeping into the uninjured side and allows the uninjured side to expand.

Recognising Rib Fractures

Rib fractures are a closed chest injury. The most common type of rib fracture is ribs fractured by a blow or a fall. The signs of a rib fracture include:

- Sharp pain, especially when casualty takes a deep breath, coughs, or moves
- Shallow breathing
- Casualty holds the injured area, trying to reduce pain

Care for Rib Fractures

To care for a rib fracture:

1. Help the casualty find the most comfortable resting position.
2. Stabilise the ribs by having the casualty hold a pillow or other similar soft object against the injured area, or use bandages to hold the pillow in place.
3. Seek medical care.

▶ Abdominal Injuries

Abdominal injuries are either open or closed. Closed abdominal injuries occur as the result of a direct blow from a blunt object. Open abdominal injuries include penetrating wounds, embedded (impaled) objects, and protruding organs.

Recognising a Closed Abdominal Injury

The signs of a closed abdominal injury include:

- Bruises or other marks
- Pain, tenderness, muscle tightness, and rigidity observed while gently pressing with your fingertips on the abdomen

Care for a Closed Abdominal Injury

To care for a closed abdominal injury:

1. Place the casualty in a comfortable position with the legs pulled up toward the abdomen.
2. Care for shock.
3. Seek medical care.

Recognising a Protruding Organ

A protruding organ injury refers to a severe injury to the abdomen in which the internal organs escape or protrude from the wound Figure 9-1A.

Care for a Protruding Organ

To care for protruding organs:

1. Place the casualty in a comfortable position with the legs pulled up toward the abdomen.
2. Cover protruding organs loosely with a moist, sterile or clean dressing Figure 9-1B.
3. Care for shock.
4. Call 9-9-9 or 1-1-2.

▶ Pelvic Injuries

Injuries to the pelvis are usually caused by a road traffic collision or a fall from a height. Pelvic fractures can be life threatening because of the large amount of blood that could be lost if the femoral artery is damaged.

Recognising Pelvic Fractures

The signs of a pelvic injury include:

- Pain in the hip, groin, or back that increases with movement
- Inability to walk or stand
- Signs of shock

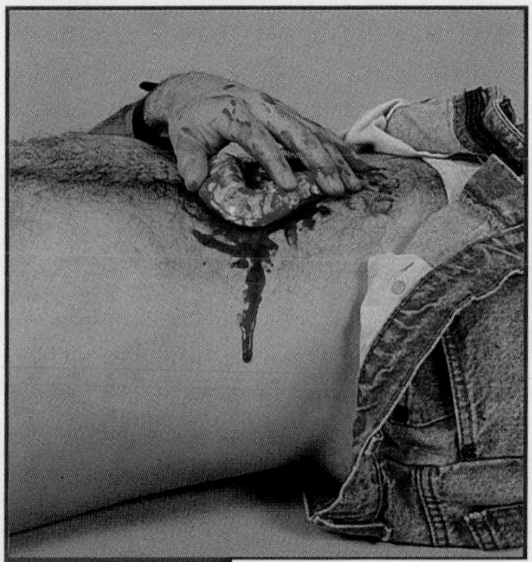

Figure 9-1A

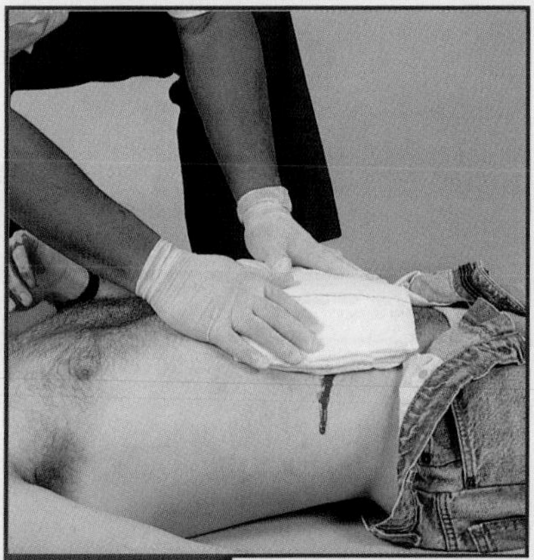

Figure 9-1B

Bandaging an open abdominal wound. **A.** Open abdominal wounds are serious injuries. **B.** Cover organs with a moist, sterile or clean dressing.

CAUTION

DO NOT try to reinsert protruding organs into the abdomen—you could introduce infection or damage the organs.

DO NOT cover the organs tightly.

DO NOT cover the organs with any material that clings or disintegrates when wet.

DO NOT give the casualty anything to eat or drink.

Care for Pelvic Fractures

To care for a pelvic injury:

1. Keep the casualty still.
2. Care for shock.
3. Call 9-9-9 or 1-1-2.

First Aid Objectives

This chapter covers the following guidelines for First Aid training and will enable the student to be able to:

- Act safely, promptly, and effectively with emergencies at work.
- Recognise the importance of personal hygiene in First Aid procedures.
- Use First Aid equipment, including the contents of a First Aid box.
- Deal with a casualty who has a chest, abdominal, or pelvic injury.

Chest Injuries

What to Look For	What to Do
Rib Fractures • Sharp pain with deep breaths, coughing, or moving • Shallow breathing • Holding of injured area to reduce pain	1. Place casualty in comfortable position. 2. Support ribs with a pillow, blanket, or coat (either holding or tying with bandages). 3. Seek medical care.

Abdominal Injuries

What to Look For	What to Do
Blow to Abdomen (Closed) • Bruise or other marks • Muscle tightness and rigidity felt while gently pushing on abdomen	1. Place casualty in comfortable position with legs pulled up towards the abdomen. 2. Care for shock. 3. Seek medical care.
Protruding Organs (Open) • Internal organs escaping from abdominal wound	1. Place casualty in a comfortable position with the legs pulled up towards the abdomen. 2. DO NOT reinsert organs into the abdomen. 3. Cover organs with a moist, sterile or clean dressing. 4. Care for shock. 5. Call 9-9-9 or 1-1-2.

Pelvic Injuries

What to Look For	What to Do
Pelvic Fractures • Pain in hip, groin, or back that increases with movement • Inability to walk or stand • Signs of shock	1. Keep casualty still. 2. Care for shock. 3. Call 9-9-9 or 1-1-2.

prep kit

▶ Key Terms

closed abdominal injuries Injuries to the abdomen that occur as a result of a direct blow from a blunt object.

closed chest injury An injury to the chest in which the skin is not broken; usually due to blunt trauma.

open abdominal injuries Injuries to the abdomen that include penetrating wounds and protruding organs.

open chest injury An injury to the chest in which the chest wall itself is penetrated, either by a fractured rib or, more frequently, by an external object such as a bullet, knife, or piece of machinery.

protruding organ injury A severe injury to the abdomen in which the internal organs escape or protrude from the wound.

▶ Assessment in Action

A 45-year-old repairman falls while carrying replacement glass for a broken window. The new glass breaks into several jagged pieces. You find the repairman lying on his back with a blood-soaked shirt. You see a lacerated abdomen with several loops of intestine protruding from the laceration.

Directions: Circle Yes if you agree with the statement, and circle No if you disagree.

Yes No 1. Gently push the protruding intestine back into the wound.

Yes No 2. Place a moist dressing over the protruding intestine.

Yes No 3. Place the casualty on his back with the knees bent.

Yes No 4. Cover the casualty with a blanket or coat.

Yes No 5. Give the casualty something to drink.

Answers: 1. No; 2. Yes; 3. Yes; 4. Yes; 5. No

▶ Check Your Knowledge

Directions: Circle Yes if you agree with the statement, and circle No if you disagree.

Yes	No	1. Stabilise a broken rib with a soft object such as a pillow or blanket tied to the chest.
Yes	No	2. Remove a penetrating or impaled object from the chest or the abdomen.
Yes	No	3. Keep the casualty with a broken pelvis still.
Yes	No	4. Sharp pain while breathing can be a sign of a rib fracture.
Yes	No	5. Rib fractures should be treated by tightly taping the chest.
Yes	No	6. Most casualties with abdominal injuries are more comfortable with their knees bent.
Yes	No	7. A broken pelvis can threaten life because of the large amount of blood lost.

Answers: **1.** Yes; **2.** No; **3.** Yes; **4.** Yes; **5.** No; **6.** Yes; **7.** Yes

10

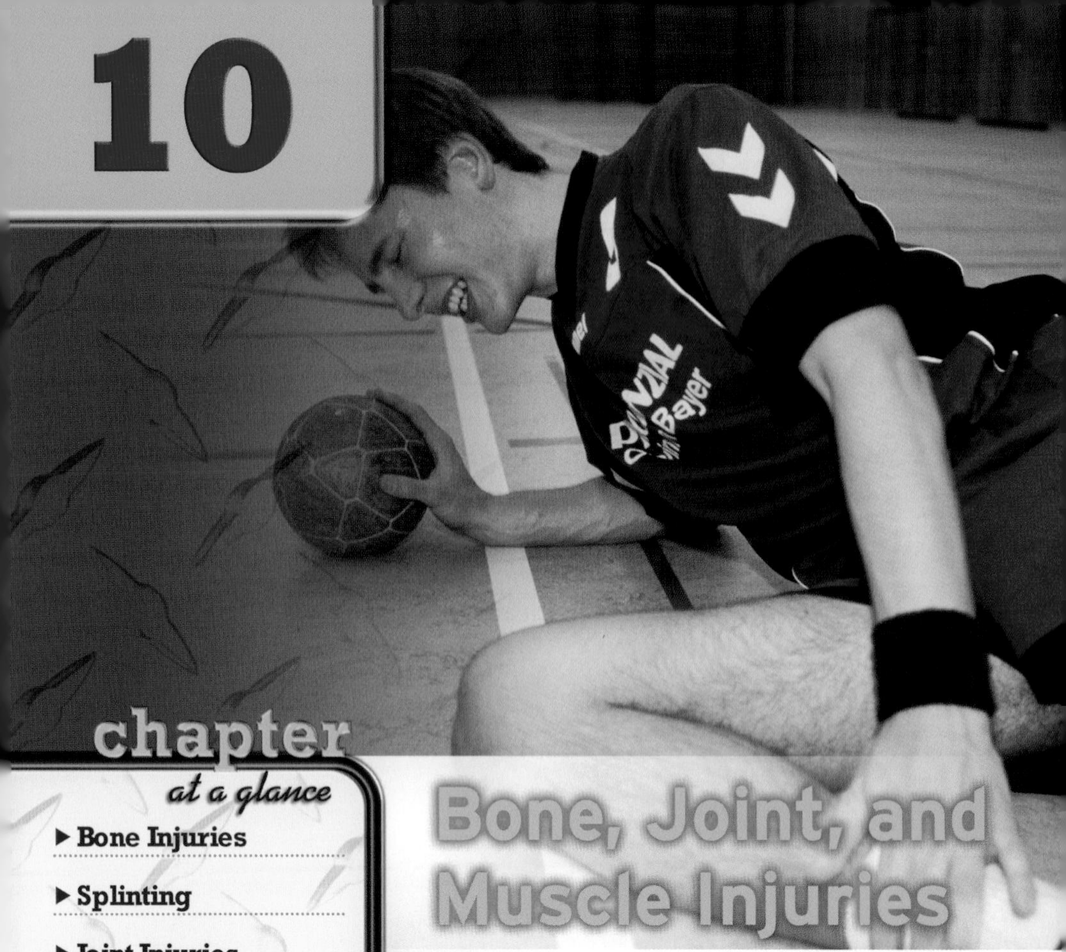

chapter *at a glance*

- Bone Injuries
- Splinting
- Joint Injuries
- RICE Procedure
- Muscle Injuries

Bone, Joint, and Muscle Injuries

▶ Bone Injuries

The terms *broken bone* and fracture have the same meaning: a break or crack in a bone. There are two categories of fractures Figure 10-1:

- Closed fracture: No open wound exists around the fracture site Figure 10-2.
- Open fracture: An open wound exists, and the broken bone end may be protruding through the skin.

Recognising Bone Injuries

It may be difficult to tell whether a bone is broken. When in doubt, provide care as if the bone were broken. Any part of the mnemonic DOTS (deformity, open wound, tenderness, swelling) can indicate a possible fracture:

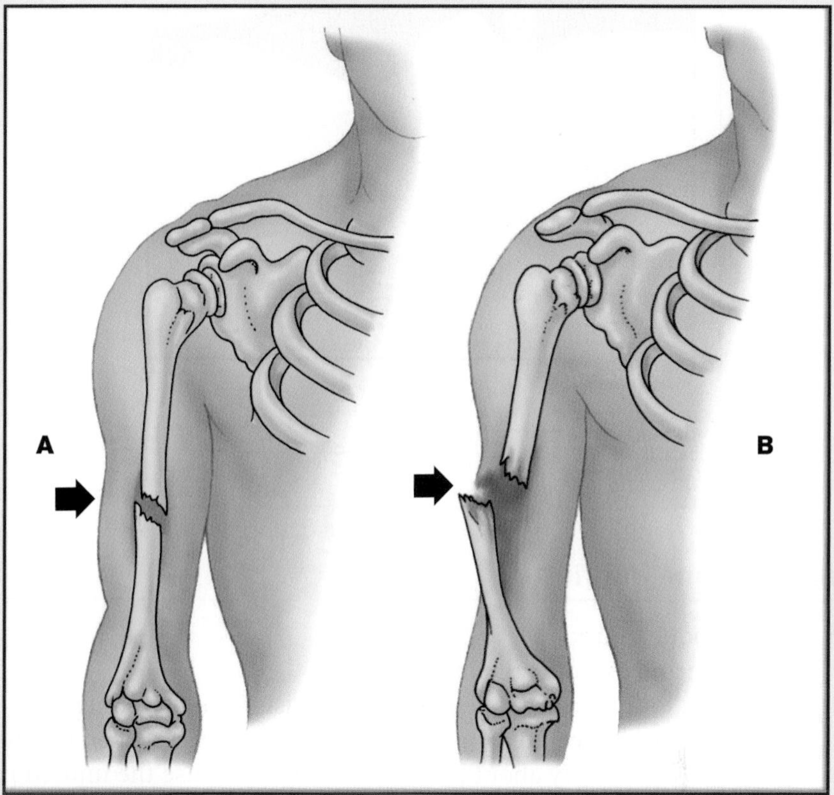

Figure 10-1

A. Closed fracture. B. Open fracture.

- *Deformity* might not be obvious. Compare the injured part with the uninjured part on the other side.
- *Open wound* may indicate an underlying fracture.
- *Tenderness* and pain are commonly found only at the injury site. The casualty can usually point to the site of the pain or feel pain when it is touched.
- *Swelling* caused by bleeding happens rapidly after a fracture.

Additional signs of a fracture include the following:

- The casualty is unable to use the injured part normally.
- A grating or grinding sensation can be felt and sometimes even heard when the ends of the broken bone rub together. This is referred to as **crepitus**.
- The casualty may have heard or felt the bone snap.

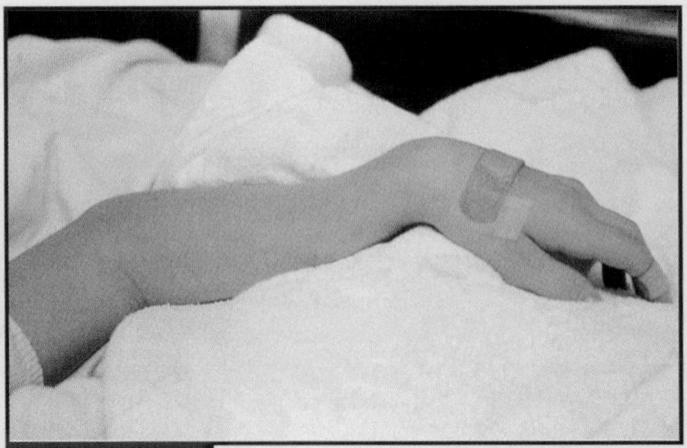

Figure 10-2

Closed forearm fracture.

Care for Bone Injuries

To care for a bone injury:

1. Expose and examine the injury site.
   - Look for deformity, open wounds, bruising, and swelling.
   - Feel the injured area for deformity and tenderness when touched.
   - Ask the casualty about pain and the ability to use the injured part normally.
2. Stabilise the injured part to prevent movement.
   - Wear appropriate protective equipment (ie, gloves, etc.).
   - If emergency medical services (EMS) will arrive soon, stabilise the injured part with your hands until they arrive.
   - If EMS will be delayed, or if you are taking the casualty to hospital, stabilise the injured part with a splint.
3. If the injury is an open fracture, do not push on any protruding bone. Cover the wound and exposed bone with a dressing. Place rolls of gauze around the bone, and bandage the injury without applying pressure on the bone.
4. Apply an ice or cold pack if possible to help reduce the swelling and pain.
5. Seek medical care. Call 9-9-9 or 1-1-2 for any open fractures or large bone fractures (such as the thigh) or when transporting the casualty would be difficult or would aggravate the injury.

▶ Splinting

Splinting an injured area helps:

- Reduce pain
- Prevent further damage to muscles, nerves, and blood vessels
- Prevent a closed fracture from becoming an open fracture
- Reduce bleeding and swelling

Splinting Guidelines

The following guidelines should be used when splinting.

- Cover any open wounds with a dry dressing before applying a splint.
- Apply a splint only if it does not cause further pain to the casualty.
- Splint the injured area in the position found.
- The splint should extend beyond the joints above and below an extremity fracture whenever possible.
- Apply splints firmly but not so tightly that blood flow to an extremity is affected.
- Elevate the injured extremity after it is splinted.
- Apply an ice or cold pack.

To splint the lower arm using a self (anatomical) splint, follow the steps in **Skill Drill 10-1**:

1. Use a triangular bandage to create a sling to support the injured arm (**Step 1**).
2. Tie the ends of the triangular bandage and secure the sling at the elbow (**Steps 2a** and **2b**).
3. Use a triangular bandage folded into a wide binder to secure the sling and the arm to the chest (**Step 3**).

To apply a rigid splint to the lower arm, follow the steps in **Skill Drill 10-2**:

1. Place a splint under the injured arm in the position found. A roll of gauze should be placed in the hand to maintain normal position of the hand (**Step 1**).
2. Secure the splint with a roll of gauze (Step 2) or two triangular bandages folded into binders.
3. Use a triangular bandage to create a sling to support the injured arm (**Step 3**).
4. Tie the ends of the triangular bandage and secure the sling at the elbow (**Step 4**).
5. Use a triangular bandage folded into a wide binder to secure the sling and the splint to the chest. (**Step 5**).

skill drill

10-1 Applying a Self (Anatomical) Splint: Lower Arm

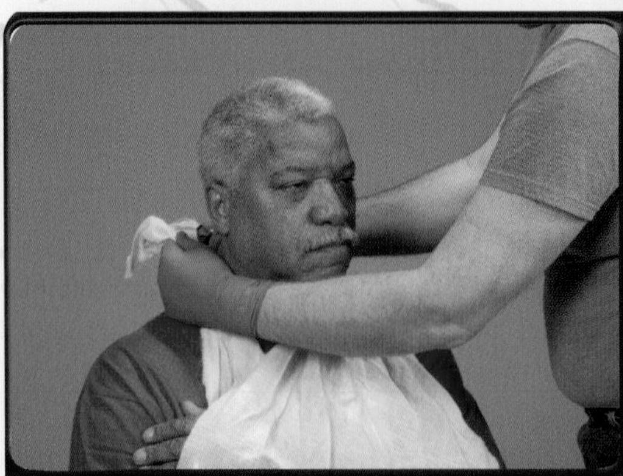

1

Use a triangular bandage to create a sling.

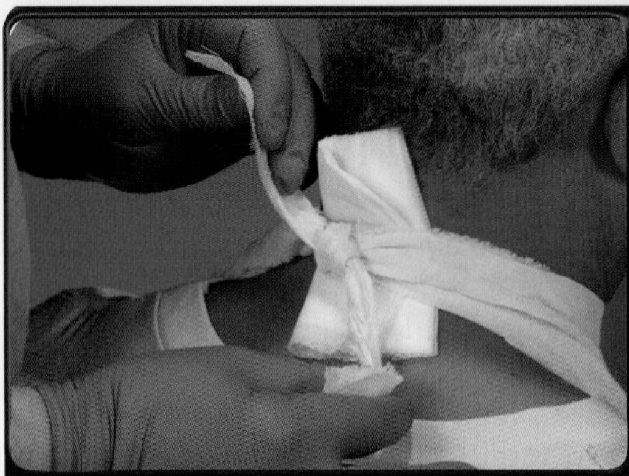

2a

Tie the ends of the triangular bandage.

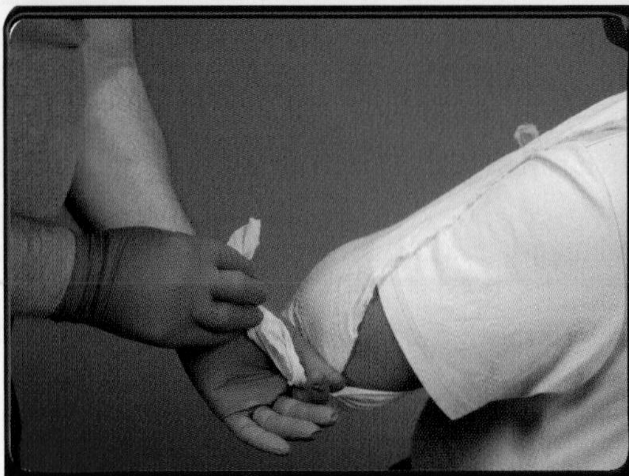

2b

Secure the sling at the elbow.

skill drill

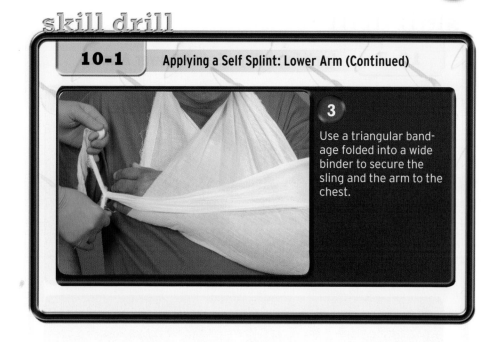

10-1 Applying a Self Splint: Lower Arm (Continued)

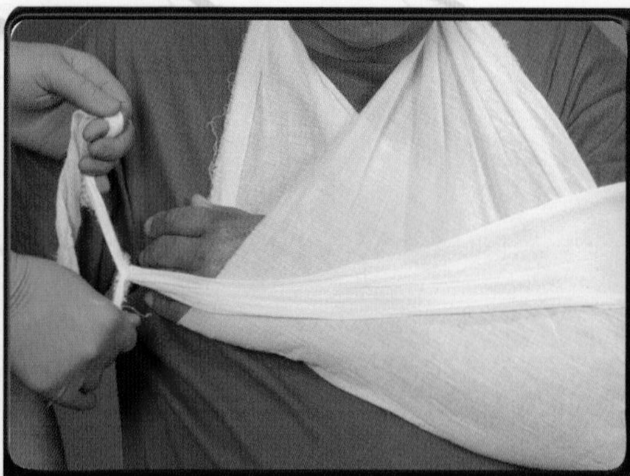

3
Use a triangular bandage folded into a wide binder to secure the sling and the arm to the chest.

To apply a soft splint to the lower arm, follow the steps in Skill Drill 10-3:

1. Use a rolled blanket or folded pillow to provide a splint for the injured arm in the position found (**Step 1**).
2. Secure the splint with several triangular bandages folded into binders (**Step 2**).
3. Use a triangular bandage to create a sling to support the injured arm (**Step 3**).
4. Tie the ends of the triangular bandage and secure the sling at the elbow (**Steps 4a** and **4b**).
5. Use a triangular bandage folded into a wide binder to secure the sling and the splint to the chest (**Step 5**).

Lower leg splints follow the same principles as lower arm splints. If more support is needed, you can bind both legs together.

▶ Joint Injuries

A sprain is a common injury to a joint in which the ligaments and other tissues are damaged by violent stretching or twisting. Attempts to move or use the joint increase the pain. Common locations for sprains include the ankles, wrists, and knees.

A dislocation is a serious and less common joint injury. It occurs when a joint comes apart and stays apart, with the bone ends no longer in contact. The shoulders, elbows, fingers, hips, knees, and ankles are the joints most frequently dislocated.

skill drill

10-2 Applying a Rigid Splint: Lower Arm

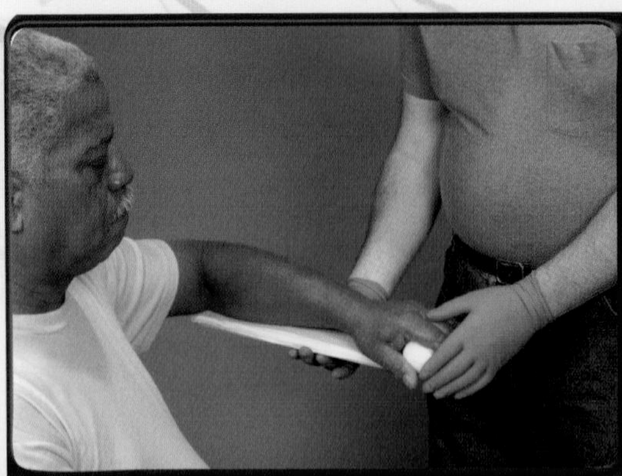

1. Place splint under the injured arm in the position found. Place hand in its normal position.

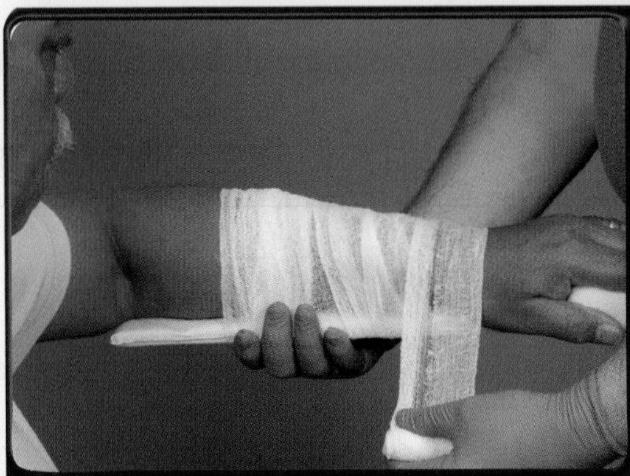

2. Secure the splint with a roll of gauze.

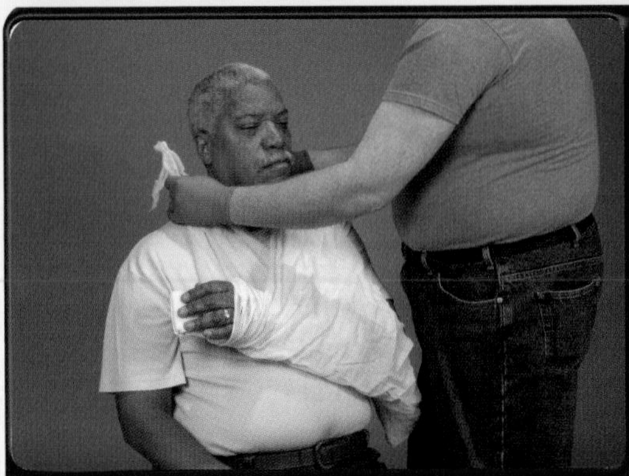

3. Create a sling using a triangular bandage.

skill drill

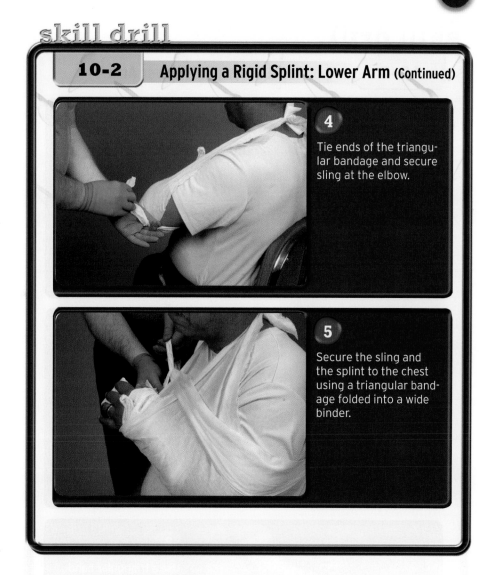

10-2 Applying a Rigid Splint: Lower Arm (Continued)

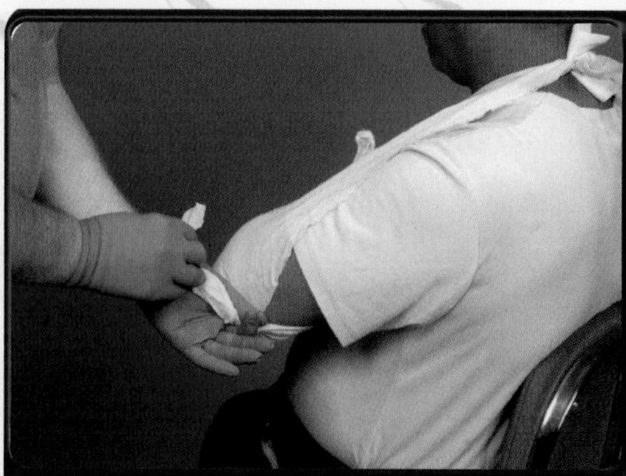

4

Tie ends of the triangular bandage and secure sling at the elbow.

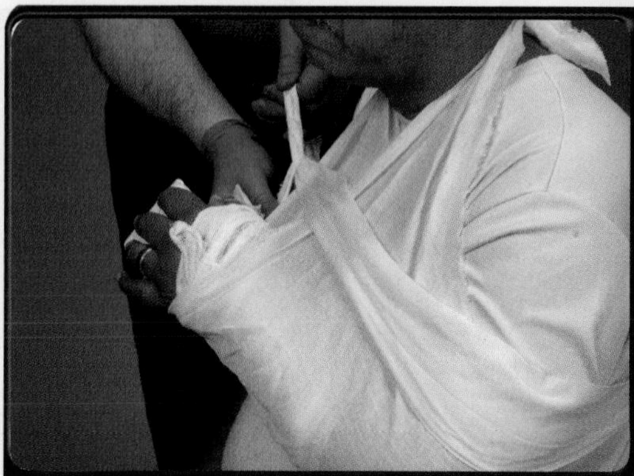

5

Secure the sling and the splint to the chest using a triangular bandage folded into a wide binder.

Recognising Joint Injuries

The signs of a sprain or dislocation are similar to those of a fracture: pain, swelling, and inability to use the injured joint normally. The main sign of a dislocation is deformity. Its appearance will be different from that of an uninjured joint Figure 10-3.

skill drill

10-3 Applying a Soft Splint: Lower Arm

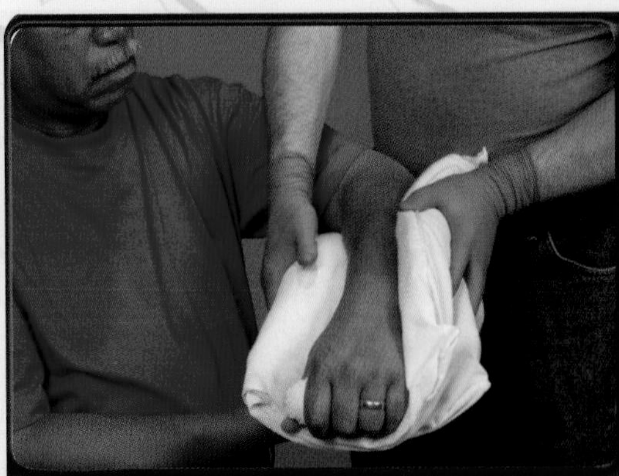

1 Use a rolled blanket or folded pillow as a splint.

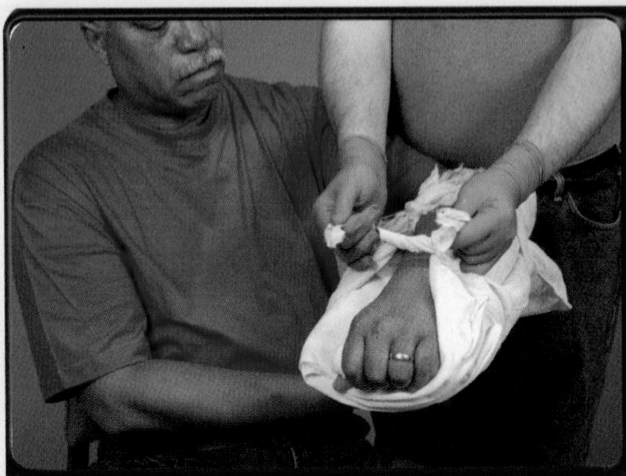

2 Secure the splint with several triangular bandages folded into binders.

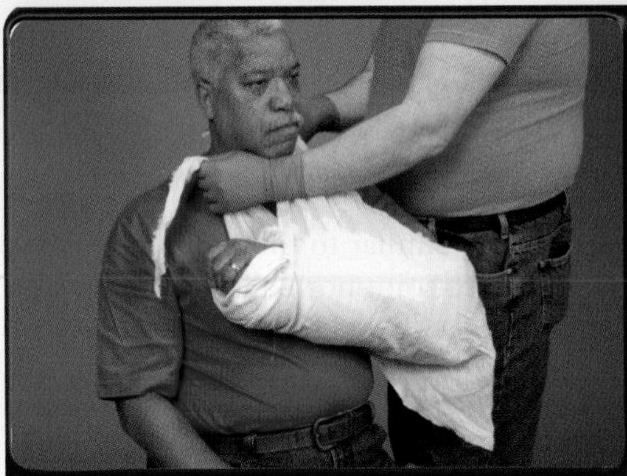

3 Use a triangular bandage to create a sling.

skill drill

10-3 Applying a Soft Splint: Lower Arm (Continued)

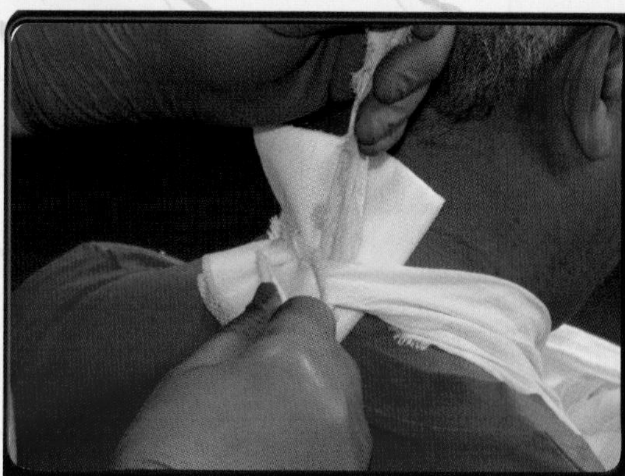

4a Tie the ends of the triangular bandage.

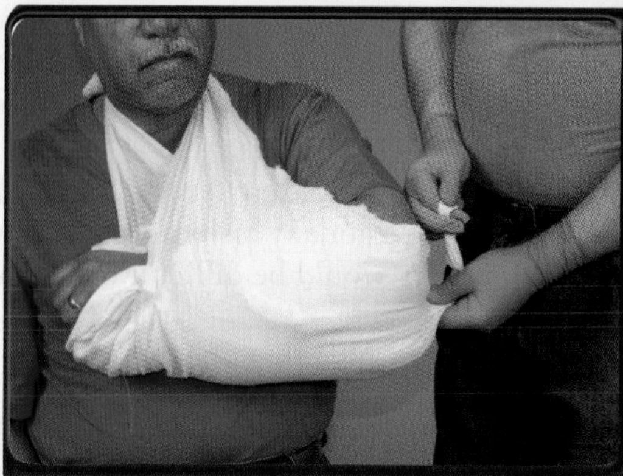

4b Secure the sling at the elbow.

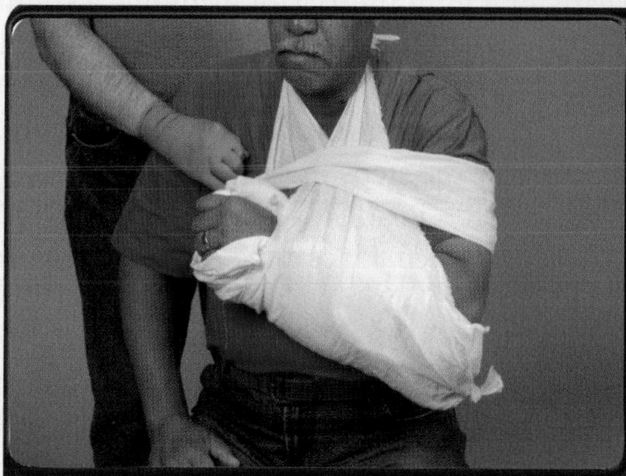

5 Use a triangular bandage folded into a wide binder to secure the sling and the splint to the chest.

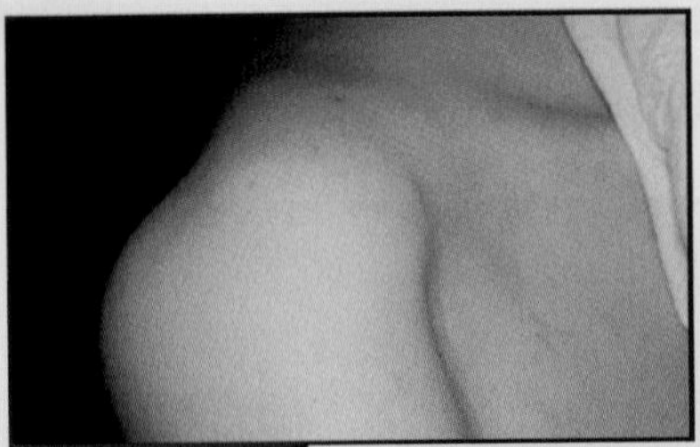
Figure 10-3A

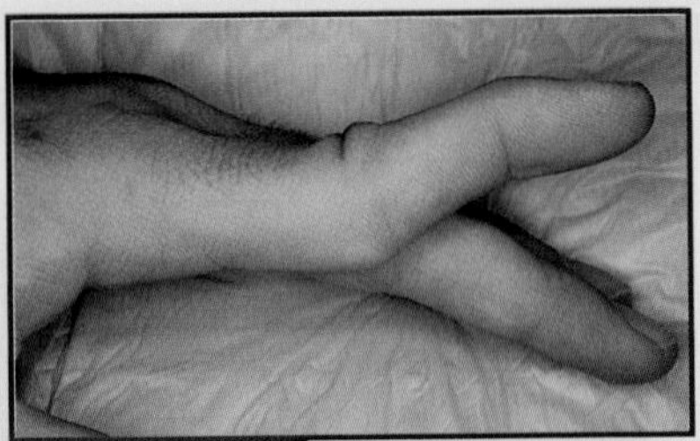
Figure 10-3B

A. Dislocated shoulder. B. Dislocated finger.

Care for Joint Injuries

To care for a joint injury:

1. If you suspect a dislocation, apply a splint if EMS will be delayed. Provide care as you would for a fracture. Do not try to put the displaced part back into its normal position, because nerve and blood vessel damage could result.
2. If you suspect a sprain, use the RICE procedure (see **Skill Drill 10-4**).
3. Seek medical care. Call 9-9-9 or 1-1-2 for any dislocations or injuries for which transporting the casualty would be difficult or would aggravate the injury.

▶ RICE Procedure

RICE is the acronym for *rest*, *ice*, *compression*, and *elevation*. This mnemonic will help you remember the care for a joint injury (for example, a sprain) or a muscle injury (for example, a strain or contusion) within the first 48 hours of it happening.

To perform the RICE procedure, follow the steps in **Skill Drill 10-4**:

1. R = Rest. Stop using the injured area.
2. I = Ice. Place an ice pack on the injured area. Use an elastic bandage to hold the ice pack in place (**Step 1**).
3. C = Compression. Remove the ice and apply a compression bandage and leave in place for 3 to 4 hours (**Step 2**).
4. E = Elevation. Raise the injured area higher than the heart, if possible (**Step 3**).

CAUTION

DO NOT apply an ice or cold pack for more than 30 minutes at a time. Frostbite or nerve damage can result.

DO NOT stop using an ice or cold pack too soon. A common mistake is the early use of heat, which increases circulation to the injured area, resulting in swelling and pain.

skill drill

10-4 RICE Procedure

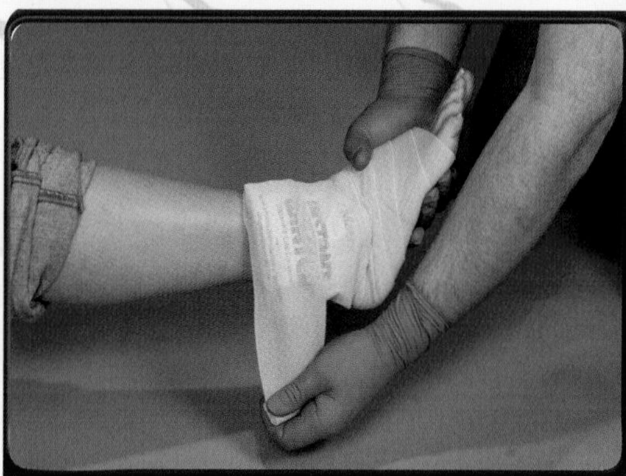

1

Place an ice pack on the injured area. Use an elastic bandage to hold the ice pack in place from between 5 and 15 minutes.

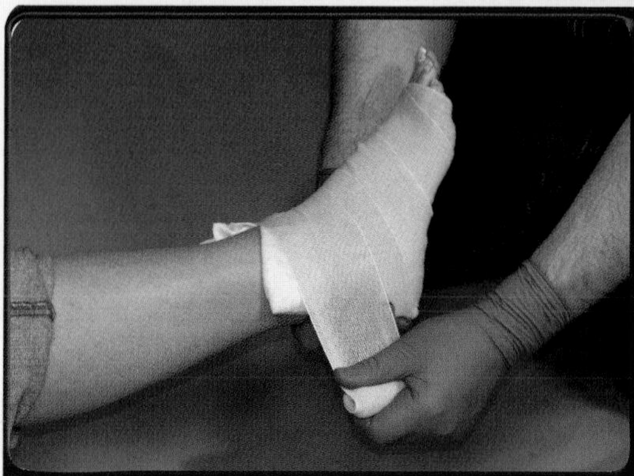

2

Remove the ice and apply a compression bandage and leave in place for 3 to 4 hours.

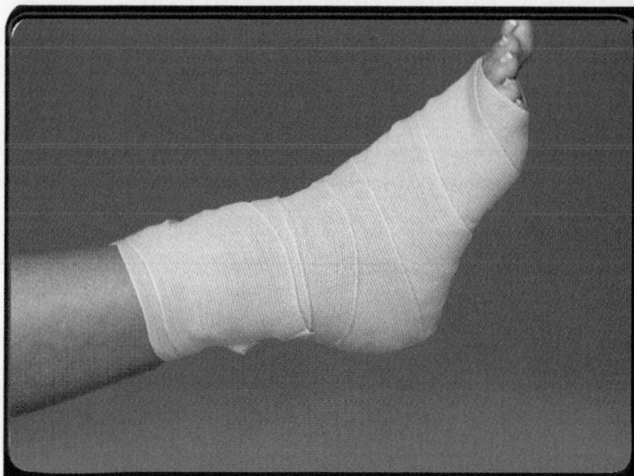

3

Raise the injured area higher than the heart, if possible.

▶ Muscle Injuries

A muscle strain, also known as a muscle pull, occurs when a muscle is overstretched and tears. Back muscles are commonly strained when people lift heavy objects.

A muscle contusion, or bruise, results from a blow to the muscle. A muscle cramp occurs when a muscle goes into an uncontrolled spasm.

Recognising Muscle Injuries

The signs of a muscle strain include the following:

- Sharp pain
- Extreme tenderness when the area is touched
- An indentation or bump that can be felt or seen
- Weakness and loss of function of the injured area
- Stiffness and pain when the casualty moves the muscle

The signs of a muscle contusion include the following:

- Pain and tenderness
- Swelling
- Bruise appearing hours after the injury

The signs of a muscle cramp include the following:

- Uncontrolled spasm
- Pain
- Restriction or loss of movement

Care for Muscle Injuries

Care for muscle strains and contusions includes resting the affected muscles and applying an ice or cold pack. To care for a muscle cramp, have the casualty stretch the affected muscle or apply pressure directly to it.

Bone, Joint, and Muscle Injuries

Type of Injury Suspected?

Bone Injury	Joint Injury	Muscle Injury
• Expose and examine the injury site. • Bandage any open wound. • Splint the injured area. • Apply an ice or cold pack. • Seek medical care.	• Expose and examine the injury site. • Splint the injured area. • Apply an ice or cold pack. • Seek medical care.	• Rest. • Apply an ice or cold pack to muscle strains and contusions. • Stretch or apply direct pressure to muscle cramps.

First Aid Objectives

This chapter covers the following guidelines for First Aid training and will enable the student to be able to:

- Act safely, promptly, and effectively with emergencies at work.
- Deal with a casualty who is suffering from an injury to bones, muscles, or joints.

Bone Injuries

What to Look For	What to Do
Fractures (Broken Bones) • DOTS (deformity, open wound, tenderness, swelling) • Inability to use injured part normally • Grating or grinding sensation felt or heard • Casualty heard or felt bone snap	1. Expose and examine the injury site. 2. Bandage any open wound. 3. Splint the injured area. 4. Apply ice or cold pack. 5. Seek medical care: Depending on the severity, call 9-9-9 or 1-1-2 or transport to medical care.

Joint Injuries

What to Look For	What to Do
Dislocation or Sprain • Deformity • Pain • Swelling • Inability to use injured part normally	**Dislocation** 1. Expose and examine the injury site. 2. Splint the injured area. 3. Apply ice or cold pack. 4. Seek medical care. **Sprain** 1. Use RICE procedures.

Muscle Injuries

What to Look For	What to Do
Strain • Sharp pain • Extreme tenderness when area is touched • Indentation or bump • Weakness and loss of function of injured area • Stiffness and pain when casualty moves the muscle	1. Use RICE procedures.
Contusion • Pain and tenderness • Swelling • Bruise on injured area	1. Use RICE procedures.
Cramp • Uncontrolled spasm • Pain • Restriction or loss of movement	1. Stretch and/or apply direct pressure to the affected muscle.

prep kit

▶ Key Terms

closed fracture A fracture in which there is no laceration in the overlying skin.

contusion A bruise; an injury that causes a haemorrhage in or beneath the skin but does not break the skin.

cramp A painful spasm, usually of a muscle.

crepitus A grating or grinding sensation that is felt and sometimes even heard when the ends of a broken bone rub together.

dislocation Bone ends at a joint are no longer in contact.

fracture Any break in a bone.

open fracture A fracture exposed to the exterior; an open wound lies over the fracture.

sling Any bandage or material that helps support the weight of an injured upper extremity.

splint A device used to stabilise an injured extremity.

sprain Torn joint ligaments.

strain Stretched or torn muscle.

▶ Assessment in Action

During a cricket match, a player bowls the ball which strikes the batsman hard on the arm. Although the skin is not broken, there is tenderness and some swelling.

Directions: Circle Yes if you agree with the statement, and circle No if you disagree.

Yes No **1.** A splint can help stabilise a broken bone against movement.

Yes No **2.** Applying heat reduces bleeding and swelling.

Yes No **3.** A splint should be applied snugly enough to reduce blood flow to the injured area.

Yes No **4.** A fracture should be splinted in the position found.

Yes No **5.** A sling can be applied after splinting an upper extremity fracture.

Answers: **1.** Yes; **2.** No; **3.** No; **4.** Yes; **5.** Yes

▶ Check Your Knowledge

Directions: Circle Yes if you agree with the statement, and circle No if you disagree.

Yes No 1. Apply cold on a suspected sprain.

Yes No 2. The letters RICE stand for rest, ice, compression, and elevation.

Yes No 3. An elastic bandage, if used correctly, can help control swelling in a joint.

Yes No 4. A broken leg can be splinted by tying both legs together.

Yes No 5. A blanket rolled around an ankle is an example of a self (anatomical) splint.

Yes No 6. A dislocation is cared for in a different way from a fracture.

Yes No 7. Check a suspected fracture by having the casualty move the extremity.

Yes No 8. Treat a muscle cramp by stretching the affected muscle.

Yes No 9. A pillow can serve as a splint.

Yes No 10. Do not push on a protruding bone.

Answers: **1.** Yes; **2.** Yes; **3.** Yes; **4.** Yes; **5.** No; **6.** No; **7.** No; **8.** Yes; **9.** Yes; **10.** Yes

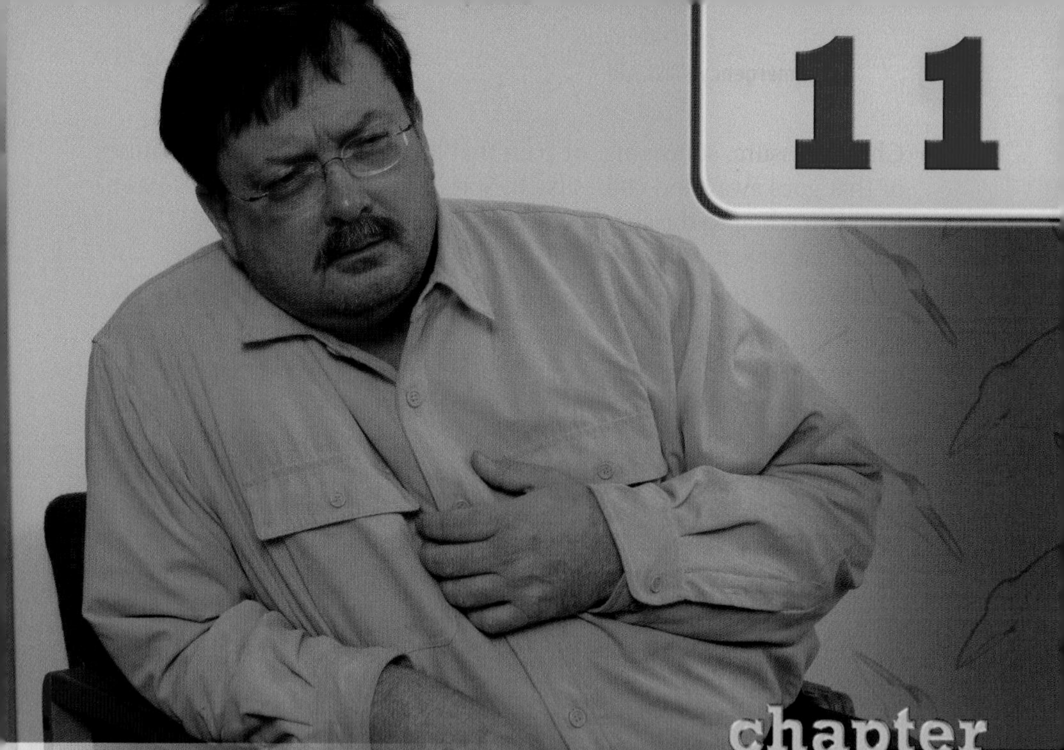

Chapter 11

Sudden Illnesses

chapter *at a glance*

- ▶ Heart Attack
- ▶ Stroke
- ▶ Breathing Difficulty
- ▶ Fainting
- ▶ Seizures
- ▶ Diabetic Emergencies

▶ Heart Attack

A heart attack occurs when the heart muscle tissue dies because its blood supply is reduced or stopped. Usually a clot in a coronary artery (the vessel that carries blood to the heart muscle) blocks the blood supply. The heart stops (known as a cardiac arrest) if a lot of the heart muscle is affected.

Recognising a Heart Attack

Prompt medical care at the onset of a heart attack is vital to survival and the quality of recovery. This is sometimes easier said than done because many casualties deny they are experiencing something as serious as a heart attack. The signs of a heart attack include the following:

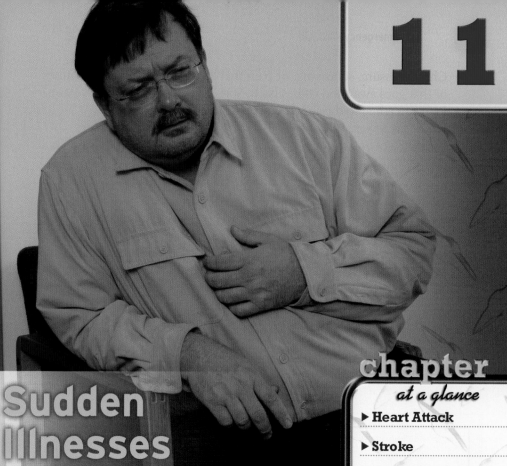

- Chest pressure, squeezing, or pain that lasts more than a few minutes or that goes away and comes back. Some patients have no chest pain.
- Pain spreading to the shoulders, neck, jaw, or arms
- Dizziness, sweating, nausea
- Shortness of breath

Care for a Heart Attack

To care for someone suffering from a potential heart attack:

1. Seek medical care by calling 9-9-9 or 1-1-2. Medications to dissolve a clot are available but must be given early.
2. Help the person into the most comfortable resting position Figure 11-1 .
3. If the casualty is alert, able to swallow, and not allergic to aspirin, give one 300 mg aspirin or two 150 mg aspirin if they are the only tablets available. The casualty should chew the tablet.
4. If the casualty has prescribed medication for heart disease, such as GTN, help the casualty use it.
5. Monitor breathing.

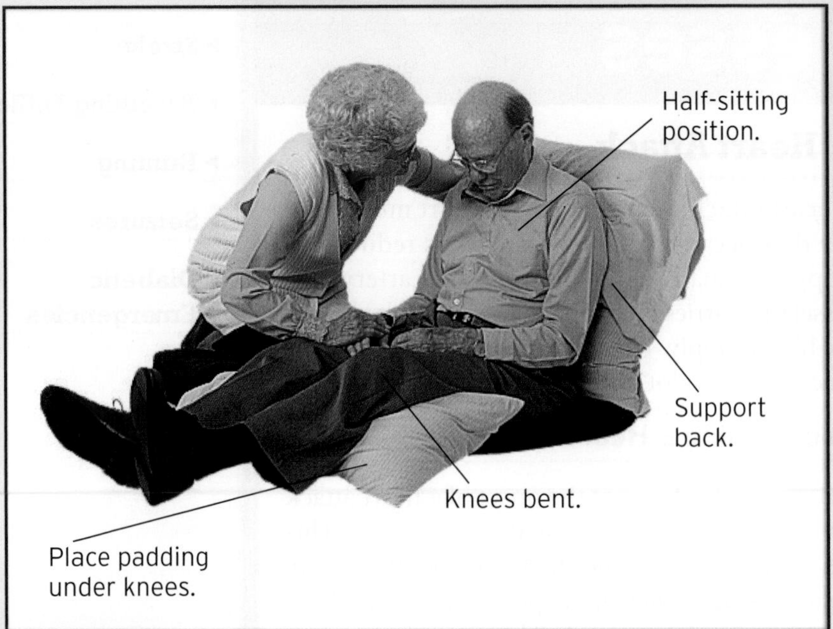
Half-sitting position.
Support back.
Knees bent.
Place padding under knees.

Figure 11-1

Help the casualty into a relaxed position to ease strain on the heart.

▶ Stroke

A stroke, also called a brain attack, occurs when part of the blood flow to the brain is suddenly cut off. This occurs when arteries in the brain rupture or become blocked.

Recognising Stroke

The signs of a stroke include the following:

- Sudden weakness or numbness of the face, an arm, or a leg on one side of the body
- Blurred or decreased vision, especially on one side of the visual field
- Problems speaking
- Dizziness or loss of balance
- Sudden, severe headache

Care for Stroke

To care for someone suffering from a stroke:

1. Call 9-9-9 or 1-1-2.
2. If the casualty is responsive, lay the casualty on his or her back with the head and shoulders slightly elevated.
3. If the casualty is unresponsive, open the airway, check breathing, and provide care accordingly. If the unresponsive casualty is breathing, place the casualty on his or her side (recovery position) to keep the airway clear.

▶ Breathing Difficulty

Asthma is a condition in which air passages narrow and mucus builds up, resulting in poor oxygen exchange. It can be triggered by such things as an allergy, cold exposure, and smoke. Hyperventilation is fast breathing, which can be caused by emotional stress, anxiety, and medical conditions.

Recognising Breathing Difficulty

The signs of breathing difficulty include the following:

- Breathing that is abnormally fast or slow
- Breathing that is abnormally deep (gasping) or shallow
- Noisy breathing, including wheezing (seen with asthma) or gurgling, crowing, or snoring sounds
- Bluish lips
- Need to pause while speaking to catch breath

Care for Breathing Difficulty

To care for a casualty with breathing difficulty:

1. Help the casualty into the most comfortable position. This is often seated upright.
2. Seek medical care by calling 9-9-9 or 1-1-2 for sudden, unknown breathing problems.
3. If the casualty has a prescribed asthma inhaler, assist the casualty in using it. If needed, the casualty may use the inhaler again in 5 to 10 minutes.
4. If the casualty's condition does not improve following inhaler use, or if the casualty's condition worsens, seek medical care by calling 9-9-9 or 1-1-2.
5. If the casualty is hyperventilating (breathing fast) due to anxiety, have him or her inhale through the nose, hold the breath for several seconds, then exhale slowly.

▶ Fainting

Fainting can happen suddenly when blood flow to the brain is interrupted. Causes include exhaustion, lack of food, reaction to pain or the sight of blood, hearing bad news, and standing too long without moving.

Recognising Fainting

The signs of fainting include the following:

- Sudden, brief unresponsiveness
- Pale skin
- Sweating

Care for Fainting

To care for fainting:

1. Open the airway, check breathing, and provide appropriate care.
2. Raise the casualty's legs, resting their feet on a chair will provide the right height.
3. Loosen any restrictive clothing.
4. If the casualty fell, check for injuries.
5. Most fainting episodes are not serious, and the casualty recovers quickly. Seek medical care if the casualty:
   - Has repeated fainting episodes
   - Does not quickly become responsive
   - Becomes unresponsive while sitting or lying down
   - Faints for no apparent reason

▶ Seizures

A seizure results from an abnormal stimulation of the brain's cells. A variety of causes can lead to seizures, including the following:

- Epilepsy
- Heatstroke
- Poisoning
- Electric shock
- Hypoglycaemia
- High fever in children
- Brain injury, tumour, or stroke
- Alcohol or other drug withdrawal or abuse

Recognising Seizure

The signs of a seizure will vary depending on the type of seizure and can include the following:

- Sudden falling
- Unresponsiveness
- Rigid body and arching of the back
- Jerky muscle movement

Care for a Seizure

To care for someone having a seizure:

1. Prevent injury by moving away any dangerous objects.
2. Loosen any restrictive clothing.
3. When the seizure is finished, place the casualty in the recovery position.
4. Call 9-9-9 or 1-1-2 if any of the following exists:
   - A seizure occurs for an unknown reason.
   - A seizure lasts more than 5 minutes.
   - The casualty is slow to recover, has a second seizure, or has difficulty breathing afterwards.
   - The casualty is pregnant or has another medical condition.
   - There are any signs of injury or illness.

CAUTION

DO NOT put anything in the casualty's mouth.
DO NOT restrain the casualty unless absolutely necessary to protect from danger.

▶ Diabetic Emergencies

Diabetes results when the body fails to produce sufficient amounts of insulin. Insulin helps regulate blood sugar level. The body cells become starved for sugar.

The body is continuously balancing sugar and insulin. Too much insulin and not enough sugar leads to low blood sugar (hypoglycaemia) and possibly insulin shock. Too much sugar and not enough insulin leads to high blood sugar (hyperglycaemia) and possibly diabetic coma.

Recognising Low Blood Sugar

A very low blood sugar level, called hypoglycaemia, can be caused by too much insulin, too little or delayed food intake, exercise, alcohol, or any combination of these factors.

In a person with diabetes, the signs of low blood sugar include the following:

- Sudden onset
- Staggering, poor coordination
- Anger, bad temper
- Pale skin
- Confusion, disorientation
- Sudden hunger
- Excessive sweating
- Trembling
- Seizures
- Unresponsiveness

Care for Low Blood Sugar

To care for a diabetic with low blood sugar (hypoglycaemia) who is responsive and can swallow:

1. Give sugar, such as two large teaspoons or lumps of sugar, a sugary drink such as regular cola or lemonade, a glass of fruit juice, a chocolate bar, or one tube of glucose gel.
2. If there is no improvement after 15 minutes, repeat giving sugar.
3. If there still is no improvement, seek medical care by calling 9-9-9 or 1-1-2.

If the victim is unresponsive, do not give anything by mouth. Call 9-9-9 or 1-1-2.

Sudden Illnesses

Type of Condition Suspected?

Stroke

- Call 9-9-9 or 1-1-2.
- If responsive, help casualty onto his or her back with head and shoulders slightly elevated.
- If unresponsive, place the casualty in the recovery position.

Breathing Difficulty

- Help casualty into a comfortable position.
- If asthma attack, help casualty with his or her prescribed inhaler medication.
- Call 9-9-9 or 1-1-2 for unknown cause or asthma not responding to inhaler treatment.
- If breathing fast (hyperventilating) due to anxiety, encourage casualty to inhale, hold breath a few seconds, then exhale.

Heart Attack

- Call 9-9-9 or 1-1-2.
- Help casualty into a comfortable position.
- Loosen any tight clothing.
- Give one 300 mg aspirin.
- Assist casualty with his or her prescribed medication.
- Monitor breathing.

Seizures

- Prevent injury.
- Loosen any tight clothing.
- Place the casualty in the recovery position.
- Call 9-9-9 or 1-1-2 if necessary.

Diabetic Emergency

If uncertain about high or low blood sugar:

- Give sugar.
- Repeat in 15 minutes.
- Call 9-9-9 or 1-1-2 if condition does not improve.

Fainting

- Check breathing.
- Check for injuries if casualty fell.
- Loosen any tight clothing.
- Raise feet onto a chair.
- Call 9-9-9 or 1-1-2 if needed.

First Aid Objectives

This chapter covers the following guidelines for First Aid training and will enable the student to be able to:

- Act safely, promptly, and effectively with emergencies at work.
- Recognise the importance of personal hygiene in First Aid procedures.
- Recognise a casualty who has a major or minor illness.

Heart Attack

What to Look For

Heart Attack
- Chest pressure, squeezing, or pain
- Pain spreading to shoulders, neck, jaw, or arms
- Dizziness, sweating, nausea
- Shortness of breath

What to Do

1. Help casualty take his or her prescribed medication.
2. Call 9-9-9 or 1-1-2.
3. Help casualty into a comfortable position.
4. Give one adult aspirin.
5. Monitor breathing.

Stroke

What to Look For

Stroke
- Sudden weakness or numbness of the face, an arm, or a leg on one side of the body
- Blurred or decreased vision
- Problems speaking
- Dizziness or loss of balance
- Sudden, severe headache

What to Do

1. Call 9-9-9 or 1-1-2.
2. If responsive, help casualty into a comfortable position with head and shoulders slightly raised.
3. If unresponsive, place the casualty in the recovery position.

Breathing Difficulty

What to Look For

Breathing Difficulty
- Abnormally fast or slow breathing
- Abnormally deep or shallow breathing
- Noisy breathing
- Bluish lips
- Need to pause while speaking to catch breath

What to Do

Unknown Reason
1. Help casualty into a comfortable position.
2. Call 9-9-9 or 1-1-2.

Asthma Attack
1. Help casualty into a comfortable position.
2. Help casualty use inhaler.
3. Call 9-9-9 or 1-1-2 if casualty does not improve.

Hyperventilating
1. Encourage casualty to inhale, hold breath a few seconds, then exhale.
2. Call 9-9-9 or 1-1-2 if condition does not improve.

Fainting

What to Look For	What to Do
Fainting • Sudden, brief unresponsiveness • Pale skin • Sweating	1. Check breathing. 2. Check for injuries if casualty fell. 3. Raise feet onto a chair. 4. Call 9-9-9 or 1-1-2 if needed.

Seizures

What to Look For	What to Do
Seizure • Sudden falling • Unresponsiveness • Rigid body and arching of back • Jerky muscle movement	1. Prevent injury. 2. Loosen any tight clothing. 3. When the seizure has finished, place the casualty in the recovery position. 4. Call 9-9-9 or 1-1-2 if needed.

Diabetic Emergencies

What to Look For	What to Do
Low Blood Sugar • Develops very quickly • Anger, bad temper • Hunger • Pale, sweaty skin	1. If uncertain about high or low sugar level, give sugar. 2. Repeat in 15 minutes if no improvement. 3. Call 9-9-9 or 1-1-2 if conditions do not improve.

prep kit

▶ Key Terms

asthma An acute spasm of the smaller air passages that causes difficult breathing and wheezing.

diabetes A disease in which the body is unable to use sugar normally because of a deficiency or total lack of insulin.

heart attack Death of a part of the heart muscle.

hyperventilation Abnormally fast breathing.

hypoglycaemia Abnormally low blood sugar level.

seizure Sudden violent muscle rigidity and jerky movements (convulsions) resulting from abnormal stimulation of the brain's cells.

stroke A blockage or rupture of arteries in the brain.

▶ Assessment in Action

A 50-year-old colleague is experiencing chest pain and nausea. He says that it started about an hour ago and has not let up. He believes it may just be indigestion. He describes the pain as "something pressing on my chest."

Directions: Circle Yes if you agree with the statement, and circle No if you disagree.

Yes No **1.** Have him lie down for 30 minutes to see if the pain subsides.

Yes No **2.** Check to see if his pupils are unequal.

Yes No **3.** His signs could indicate a heart attack.

Yes No **4.** Help the casualty take an aspirin, and call EMS.

Yes No **5.** Heart attack victims often resist the idea that they need medical care.

Answers: **1.** No; **2.** No; **3.** Yes; **4.** Yes; **5.** Yes

▶ Check Your Knowledge

Directions: Circle Yes if you agree with the statement, and circle No if you disagree.

Yes No **1.** Heart attack victims can experience chest pain.

Yes No **2.** You can encourage someone who is suffering from chest pain to take their GTN.

Yes No **3.** A responsive stroke casualty should lie down with his or her head slightly raised.

Yes No **4.** People with asthma may have a prescribed inhaler.

Yes No **5.** A casualty who is breathing fast (hyperventilation) should be encouraged to breathe slowly by holding inhaled air for several seconds and then exhaling slowly.

Yes No **6.** Raise the feet of a person who has fainted up onto seat level of a chair.

Yes No **7.** Some seizure casualties display a rigid arching of the back.

Yes No **8.** A person having seizures always requires medical attention.

Yes No **9.** If in doubt about the type of diabetic emergency a person is experiencing, give sugar to a responsive casualty who can swallow.

Answers: **1.** Yes; **2.** Yes; **3.** Yes; **4.** Yes; **5.** Yes; **6.** Yes; **7.** Yes; **8.** No; **9.** Yes

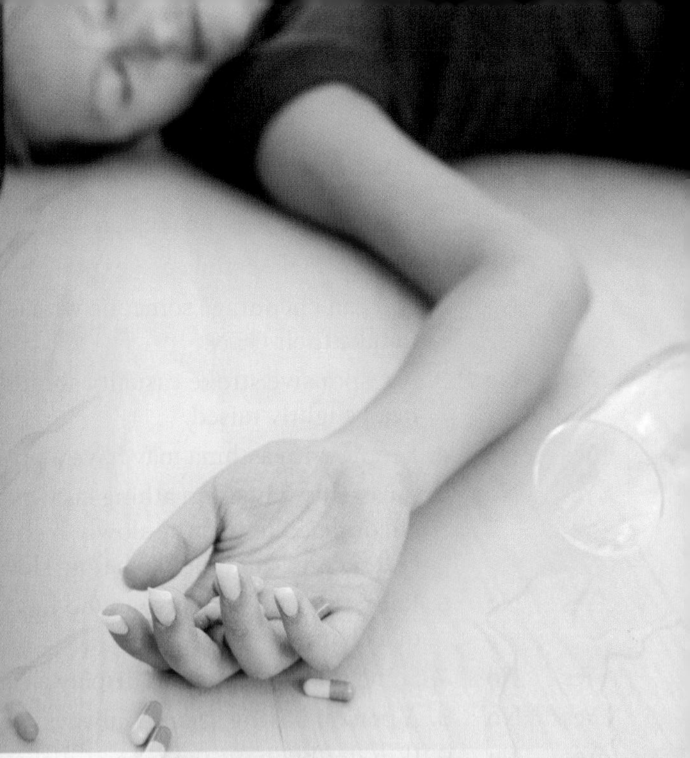

12

chapter

at a glance

▸ Poisons

▸ Ingested Poisons

Poisoning

▸ Poisons

A <u>poison</u> is any substance that impairs health or causes death by its chemical action when it enters the body or comes in contact with the skin.

▸ Ingested Poisons

<u>Ingested poisoning</u> occurs when the casualty swallows a toxic substance. Fortunately, most poisons have little toxic effect or are ingested in such small amounts that severe poisoning rarely occurs. However, the potential for severe or fatal poisoning is always present. About 80% of all poisonings happen because of ingestion of a toxic substance.

Recognising Ingested Poisoning

The signs of ingested poisoning include the following:

- Abdominal pain and cramping
- Nausea or vomiting
- Diarrhoea
- Burns, odour, or stains around and in the mouth
- Drowsiness or unresponsiveness
- Poison container nearby

Care for Ingested Poisons

To care for someone who has ingested poisons:

1. Determine the following:
   - The age and size of the casualty
   - What was swallowed (read container label; save vomit for analysis)
   - How much was swallowed (for example, a dozen tablets)
   - When it was swallowed
2. If the casualty is responsive:
   - Ask them what they have swallowed.
   - Try to reassure them.
   - Dial 9-9-9 or 1-1-2 for an ambulance.
   - Give as much information as possible about the swallowed poison. This information will assist doctors to give appropriate treatment once the casualty reaches hospital.
3. If the casualty is unresponsive:
   - Open the airway and check breathing.
   - If required, perform chest compressions and rescue breaths. Extreme caution must be used when giving rescue breaths to a casualty who is possibly contaminated. If possible, use a face shield or similar device. If nothing is available and you are unsure, it is acceptable to perform compression-only resuscitation.
   - If the casualty is unconscious but breathing normally, place the casualty in the recovery position. It is preferable to place the casualty on his or her left side to delay absorption of the poison and to prevent aspiration (inhalation) into the lungs if vomiting begins Figure 12-1.

CAUTION

DO NOT give water or milk to dilute poisons unless instructed to do so by a medical adviser.

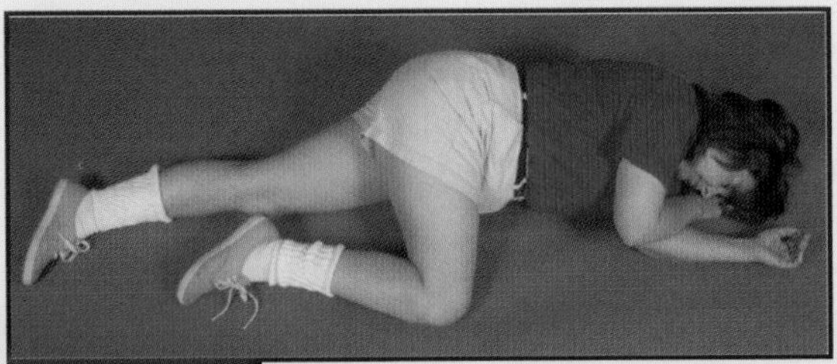

Figure 12-1

The left-side position delays a poison's absorption into the casualty's circulatory system.

Ingested Poison

Responsive or Unresponsive Casualty?

Responsive Casualty

- Reassure the casualty.
- Dial 9-9-9 or 1-1-2 for an ambulance.
- Collect as much information as possible about the poison.

Unresponsive Casualty

- Open airway, check breathing, and treat accordingly.
- If breathing, place the casualty on the left side.
- Call 9-9-9 or 1-1-2.

First Aid Objectives

This chapter covers the following guidelines for First Aid training and will enable the student to be able to:

- Act safely, promptly, and effectively with emergencies at work.
- Deal with a casualty who has been poisoned or exposed to a harmful substance.

Poisoning

What to Look For

Ingested (Swallowed) Poisoning

- Abdominal pain and cramping
- Nausea or vomiting
- Diarrhoea
- Burns, odour, or stains around and in mouth
- Drowsiness or unresponsiveness
- Poison container nearby

What to Do

1. Determine the age and size of the casualty, what and how much was swallowed, and when it was swallowed.
2. If the casualty is responsive, reassure the casualty. Dial 9-9-9 or 1-1-2 for an ambulance and try to collect as much information as possible about the poison.
3. If casualty is unresponsive, open airway, check breathing, and treat accordingly. If breathing, place on left side in recovery position. Call 9-9-9 or 1-1-2.

prep kit

▶ Key Terms

<u>ingested poisoning</u> Poisoning caused by swallowing a toxic substance.

<u>poison</u> Any substance that impairs health or causes death by its chemical action when it enters the body or comes in contact with the skin; also known as a toxin.

▶ Assessment in Action

You find your 2-year-old son vomiting. You notice that the top of a nearby medicine bottle is off. The label on the bottle reveals that the medicine inside belongs to your mother, who is visiting. You realise that he must have swallowed some of the highly potent medicine.

Directions: Circle Yes if you agree with the statement, and circle No if you disagree.

Yes No **1.** Immediately have him drink water or milk.

Yes No **2.** Call the poison control centre immediately.

Yes No **3.** Induce vomiting.

Yes No **4.** Place him on his left side.

Yes No **5.** Attempt to collect information such as the type of medicine taken, how many pills were left in the bottle, etc.

Answers: **1.** No; **2.** No; **3.** No; **4.** Yes; **5.** Yes

▶ Check Your Knowledge

Directions: Circle Yes if you agree with the statement, and circle No if you disagree.

Yes No **1.** Swallowing a poison can produce nausea.

Yes No **2.** Activated charcoal can be used for all casualties of ingested poison.

Yes No **3.** Vomit can be thrown/flushed away as it is not important to retain samples.

Yes No **4.** Causing a poisoned casualty to vomit is a recommended first aid practice.

Answers: **1.** Yes; **2.** No; **3.** No; **4.** No

glossary

A

abandonment Failure to continue first aid until relieved by someone with the same or higher level of training.

adrenaline auto-injector Prescribed device used to administer an emergency dose of adrenaline to a casualty experiencing anaphylaxis.

airborne diseases Infections transmitted through the air, such as tuberculosis.

airway obstruction A blockage, often the result of a foreign body, in which air flow to the lungs is reduced or completely blocked.

anaphylaxis A life-threatening allergic reaction.

anterior nosebleed Bleeding from the front of the nose.

arterial bleeding Bleeding from an artery; this type of bleeding tends to spurt with each heartbeat.

asthma An acute spasm of the smaller air passages that causes difficult breathing and wheezing.

B

bandage Used to cover a dressing to keep it in place on the wound and to apply pressure to help control bleeding.

bloodborne diseases Infections transmitted through the blood, such as HIV or hepatitis B virus.

C

capillary bleeding Bleeding that oozes from a wound steadily but slowly.

cardiac arrest Stoppage of the heartbeat.

cardiopulmonary resuscitation (CPR) The act of providing rescue breaths and chest compressions for a casualty in cardiac arrest.

chain of survival A four-step concept to help improve survival from cardiac arrest: early access, early CPR, early defibrillation, and early advanced care.

chest compressions Depressing the chest and allowing it to return to its normal position as part of CPR.

closed abdominal injuries Injuries to the abdomen that occur as a result of a direct blow from a blunt object.

closed chest injury An injury to the chest in which the skin is not broken; usually due to blunt trauma.

closed fracture A fracture in which there is no laceration in the overlying skin.

concussion A temporary disturbance of brain activity caused by a blow to the head.

consent Permission from a casualty to allow the first aider to provide care.

contusion A bruise; an injury that causes a haemorrhage in or beneath the skin but does not break the skin.

cramp A painful spasm, usually of a muscle.

crepitus A grating or grinding sensation that is felt and sometimes even heard when the ends of a broken bone rub together.

cyanosis Low levels of oxygen in the blood that result in the skin and mucous membranes becoming blue or grey.

D

diabetes A disease in which the body is unable to use sugar normally because of a deficiency or total lack of insulin.

dislocation Bone ends at a joint are no longer in contact.

DOTS The mnemonic for remembering key signs of a problem: *Deformities*, *Open wounds*, *Tenderness*, and *Swelling*.

dressing A sterile gauze pad or clean cloth covering placed over an open wound.

duty of care An individual's responsibility to ensure that any treatment they may provide is in accordance with the training they have taken and within their expertise.

E

expressed consent Consent explicitly given by a casualty that permits the first aider to provide care.

F

first aid Immediate care given to an injured or suddenly ill person.

flail chest A condition that occurs when several ribs in the same area are broken in more than one place.

fracture Any break in a bone.

full-thickness burn A burn that penetrates all the skin layers into the underlying fat and muscle.

H

haemorrhage A large amount of bleeding in a short time.

heart attack Death of a part of the heart muscle.

hepatitis A viral infection of the liver.

human immunodeficiency virus (HIV) The virus that causes acquired immunodeficiency syndrome (AIDS).

hyperventilation Abnormally fast breathing.

hypoglycaemia Abnormally low blood sugar level.

I

implied consent Consent assumed because the casualty is unresponsive, mentally incompetent, or underage and has no parent or guardian present.

ingested poisoning Poisoning caused by swallowing a toxic substance.

initial check The first step in dealing with an emergency situation; this step determines whether there are life-threatening problems requiring quick care.

M

medical identification tag A bracelet or necklace that notes the wearer's medical problem(s) and a 24-hour telephone number for emergency access to the casualty's medical history plus names of doctors and close relatives.

N

negligence Deviation from the accepted standard of care resulting in further injury to the casualty.

O

open abdominal injuries Injuries to the abdomen that include penetrating wounds and protruding organs.

open chest injury An injury to the chest in which the chest wall itself is penetrated, either by a fractured rib or, more frequently, by an external object such as a bullet, knife, or piece of machinery.

open fracture A fracture exposed to the exterior; an open wound lies over the fracture.

P

partial-thickness burn A burn that extends through the skin's entire outer layer and into the inner layer.

personal protective equipment (PPE) Equipment, such as medical examining gloves, used to block the entry of an organism into the body.

physical examination Process of gathering information about the casualty's condition by noting the casualty's signs.

poison Any substance that impairs health or causes death by its chemical action when it enters the body or comes in contact with the skin; also known as a toxin.

posterior nosebleed Bleeding from the back of the nose into the mouth or down the back of the throat.

protruding organ injury A severe injury to the abdomen in which the internal organs escape or protrude from the wound.

R

rescue breaths Breathing for a person who is not breathing.

S

SAMPLE The mnemonic for remembering key information about a patient's history: *Symptoms*, *Allergies*, *Medications*, *Past* medical history, *Last* oral intake, and *Events* leading up to the injury or illness.

scene size-up Quick survey of an emergency scene to determine whether there are life-threatening problems requiring quick care.

seizure Sudden violent muscle rigidity and jerky movements (convulsions) resulting from abnormal stimulation of the brain's cells.

shock Inadequate tissue oxygenation resulting from serious injury or illness.

skull fracture A break of part of the skull (head bones).

sling Any bandage or material that helps support the weight of an injured upper extremity.

splint A device used to stabilise an injured extremity.

sprain Torn joint ligaments.

strain Stretched or torn muscle.

stroke A blockage or rupture of arteries in the brain.

sucking chest wound A chest wound that allows air to pass into and out of the chest cavity with each breath.

superficial burn A burn that affects the skin's outer layer.

T

tuberculosis (TB) A bacterial disease that usually affects the lungs.

V

venous bleeding Bleeding from a vein; this type of bleeding tends to flow steadily.

index

9-9-9 or 1-1-2 calls
and abdominal injuries, 93
and amputations, 56
and anaphylaxis, 64, 66
and bleeding, 55, 59
and bone injuries, 98, 110
and breathing difficulties, 115, 119, 120
and burns, 72
and heart attacks, 30, 114, 119, 120
and hypoglycaemia, 118, 121
and initial physical examination, 9–11
and internal bleeding, 56
and joint injuries, 106
and pelvic injuries, 92, 93
and poisoning, 125, 126, 127
and seizures, 117, 119, 121
and spinal injuries, 84, 86
and strokes, 115, 119, 120

A

abandonment, 4, 6
abdominal injuries, 90–91, 93
abdominal pain or pressure, 10, 125, 127
abdominal thrusts for choking, 46
adrenaline auto-injector, 64–65, 67
agitation, 63
airborne diseases, 12, 14
airway obstruction, 39–48
    and anaphylaxis, 63
    and CPR, 31–32, 35, 38, 40–41
    definition, 48
    and electrical burns, 74
    and initial physical examination, 17, 18–19, 21, 22
    and vomiting, 55
alcohol abuse and seizures, 117
amputations, 56
anaphylaxis, 63–67
animal bites, 10
anterior nosebleeds, 82, 87
anxiety, 63, 66, 115, 116, 119
arterial bleeding, 51, 60
aspirin and heart attacks, 114, 119, 120
asthma, 115, 119, 122

B

back blows and choking, 41–46
bandages, 57–58, 60
bites, 10
bleeding
  and bandages, 57–59
  external, 50–53, 59
  and fractures, 97, 99
  and head wounds, 76–77, 78, 85
  initial physical examination, 17, 18, 19
  internal, 52–55, 59
  and nosebleeds, 82–83, 86
  and open wounds, 20, 50–53, 55, 59
  overview, 59
  unstoppable, 10
blood sugar, low (hypoglycaemia), 117, 118, 121
bloodborne disease, 11–12, 14
bone injuries, 90–92, 96–101, 109
brain injuries, 78–79, 117. *See also* strokes
breathing difficulties, 10, 115–16, 119, 120. *See also* airway obstruction; CPR
  abnormal sounds, 20
  and anaphylaxis, 64, 66
  and heart attacks, 114, 120
  initial physical examination, 17, 19
  shortness of breath, 10, 64, 114, 120
broken bones. *See* bone injuries
bruises and bruising, 52, 54, 59, 90, 93, 108–9, 110
burns, 10, 69–75, 125, 127

C

capillary bleeding, 50, 60
cardiac arrest, 29–39, 48
cardiopulmonary resuscitation. *See* CPR
cardiovascular disease, 30
chain of survival, 30, 48
chemical burns, 72, 74
chemicals in the eye, 81, 85
chest compression, 33, 48
chest injuries, 89–90, 93
chest pain or pressure, 10, 114, 120
children
  and CPR, 35, 38–39, 43
  and seizures, 117
choking, 41–47
closed abdominal injuries, 90, 94
closed chest injuries, 89, 94
closed fractures, 96–97, 111. *See also* bone injuries
compression
  and internal bleeding, 54, 59
  and joint injuries, 106–7
  and muscle injuries, 110
compression-only CPR, 41
concussion, 78, 87
confusion, 63, 118
consciousness, loss of, 10, 79. *See also* responsiveness
consent, 4, 6
contusions, 108, 111
coughing and anaphylaxis, 63, 66

CPR
- and breathing difficulties, 42–44
- and children, 35, 38–39, 43
- definition, 48
- and heart attacks, 30
- and infants, 37, 40–41, 43
- overview, 47
- performing, 13, 31–39

cramps, muscle, 108–111
crepitus, 97, 111
cyanosis, 24, 27

D

dazed behaviour, 10, 79
defibrillation, 30, 31
deformities, 10
- and bone injuries, 97, 98, 110
- and dislocations, 103
- and head injuries, 77, 85
- and initial physical examination, 20, 21
- and joint injuries, 110
- and spinal injuries, 83
- and sprains, 103

diabetes, 118, 119, 121, 122
diarrhoea and poisoning, 127
direct pressure to control bleeding, 51–53
disease transmission, 11–13
dislocations, 101, 103, 106, 111
disorientation, 118

dizziness, 10
and anaphylaxis, 64, 66
and brain injuries, 79, 85
and heart attacks, 114, 120
and strokes, 115, 120
documentation, 5
DOTS (deformity, open wound, tenderness, swelling), 20–24, 27, 96–97, 110
dressings, 57, 60
drowsiness, 79, 125, 127
drug abuse and seizures, 117
drug overdose, 10
duty of care, 4, 6

E

electrical burns, 72–73, 74
electrical shock, 117
elevation
and joint injuries, 106–7
and muscle injuries, 110
of wounds, 51, 53, 55
embedded objects, 51, 77, 81
emergencies, 8–15
Emergency Medical Services (EMS), 9
epilepsy, 117
expressed consent, 4, 6
eye injuries, 51, 79–81, 85

F

face, injuries to, 10, 115, 120
fainting, 10, 116, 119, 121
falling and seizures, 117, 121
fever, 10, 117
first aid, definition, 6
first aid kits, 1, 3
flail chest, 94
fontanelle, 10
foreign bodies, 10
fractures. *See* bone injuries
full-thickness burns, 70, 72, 74, 75

G

gloves, 12, 13, 51–52
Good Samaritan laws, 4

H

haemorrhage, 50, 60
hallucinations, 10
handover of casualty, 26
hands, deep cuts on, 10
head injuries, 10, 21, 22, 76–83, 85
headaches, 10, 79, 85, 115, 120

Health and Safety (First Aid) Regulations 1981, 2
heart attacks, 29–39, 48, 113–14, 119, 120, 122
heatstroke, 117
hepatitis, 11–12, 14
history of illness or injury, 24–25
homicidal feelings, 10
human immunodeficiency virus (HIV), 12, 14
hunger and hypoglycaemia, 118
hyperventilation, 115, 119, 120, 122
hypoglycaemia, 117, 118, 121, 122

I

ice
    and bone injuries, 98, 99, 109, 110
    and internal bleeding, 54, 59
    and joint injuries, 106–7, 109, 110
    and muscle injuries, 108–9, 110

implied consent, 4, 6
infants
    and choking, 43, 46
    and CPR, 32, 37, 40–41

ingested poisoning, 124, 128
inhalers, 115, 119
initial physical examination, 17–24, 27
injuries, 1–2, 10. *See also* specific type of injury
internal bleeding, 52–55, 59
itching and anaphylaxis, 64

J

joint injuries, 101, 103, 106, 109, 110

K

kits, first aid, 1

L

laws and first aid, 2–3, 4
loss of consciousness, 10, 79. *See also* responsiveness
low blood sugar (hypoglycaemia), 117, 118, 121

M

medical identification tag, 24, 27
medications, 3. *See also* aspirin and heart attacks; inhalers
mood changes, 79, 85
mouth-to-barrier device, 33–34
mouth-to-mouth rescue breathing, 33–34. *See also* CPR
mouth-to-nose rescue breathing, 33–34. *See also* CPR
mouth-to-stoma rescue breathing, 33–34. *See also* CPR
muscle injuries, 108–9

N

nausea
 and anaphylaxis, 64, 66
 and brain injuries, 79, 85
 and heart attacks, 114, 120
 and poisoning, 125, 127
 and shock, 63, 66
neck stiffness, 10
negligence, 4, 6
nose injuries, 82–83, 86
nosebleeds, 82–83
numbness in limbs, 83, 86, 115, 120

O

open abdominal injuries, 90–91, 94
open chest injuries, 89, 94
open fractures, 96–97, 111. *See also* bone injuries
open wounds, 20, 21, 50–53, 55, 59. *See also* open abdominal injuries; open chest injuries
organs, protruding, 91, 94
overdose, drug, 10

P

pain
 and abdominal injuries, 90
 abdominal pain or pressure, 10
 and broken nose, 83, 86
 and burns, 69–71, 74
 chest pain or pressure, 10, 114, 120

and fractures, 77, 85, 90, 91, 93, 97–98
and heart attacks, 114, 120
and internal bleeding, 54, 59
and joint injuries, 101, 103, 110
and muscle injuries, 108–9, 110
and poisoning, 125, 127
and spinal injuries, 83, 86
and splinting, 99
sudden and severe, 10
partial-thickness burns, 69–70, 71–72, 74, 75
pelvic injuries, 91–92, 93
personal protective equipment (PPE), 12, 14
physical examination, 19, 21–24, 27
poisons and poisoning, 10, 117, 124–28
posterior nosebleeds, 82, 87
pressure points, 52, 54
protruding organ injuries, 91, 94
puncture wounds, 10
pupil size, 10, 21, 22, 79, 85

R

recovery position, 25, 26, 42, 65, 66, 115
Reporting of Injuries, Diseases, and Dangerous Occurrences Regulations, 3–4
rescue breaths, 33–34, 48. *See also* CPR
responsiveness, 117
and airway obstruction, 17, 19, 39, 42–43
and brain injuries, 85
and CPR, 31, 35, 37, 43, 47
and fainting, 116, 121
and head injuries, 31, 85
and hypoglycaemia, 118

responsiveness (*continued*)
and implied consent, 64
and initial physical examination, 17, 18
and poisoning, 125, 127
and seizures, 117, 121
and shock, 63, 65, 66

rest, 54, 59, 106–7
restlessness, 63, 66
rib fractures, 90
RICE (rest, ice, compression, and elevation), 54–55, 59, 106–7, 110
rigidity, 90, 93, 117, 121
risk factors of cardiovascular disease, 30

S

SAMPLE (medical history), 24–25, 27
scalp wounds, 76–77
scene size-up, 9, 16, 27
seizures, 117–119, 121, 122
shock, 62–67
and abdominal injuries, 90, 93
and amputations, 56
and internal bleeding, 54, 55, 59
and pelvic injuries, 91–93
and skin changes, 63

shortness of breath, 10, 64, 114, 120
skin changes
and airway obstruction, 39
and anaphylaxis, 64, 66

skin changes (*continued*)
  and fainting, 116, 121
  initial primary evaluation, 24
  and hypoglycaemia, 118
  and shock, 63, 66
skull fractures, 51, 77–78, 87
slings, 99–105, 111
sneezing and anaphylaxis, 63, 66
speech difficulties, 115, 120
spinal injuries, 20, 83–84, 86
splints and splinting, 98, 99–105, 106, 109–111
sprains, 101, 103, 111
stoma rescue breathing, 33–34
stomach distension, 34
stool, blood in, 54
strains, 108, 111
strokes, 115, 117, 119, 122
stupor, 10
sucking chest wound, 94
suicidal feelings, 10
superficial burns, 69, 70, 71, 74, 75
supplies, first aid, 1, 3
sweating, 114, 116, 118, 120, 121
swelling
  and anaphylaxis, 64
  and bone injuries, 97, 110
  and initial physical examination, 20, 21
  and joint injuries, 110
  and muscle injuries, 108–9
  and sprains, 103

T

tenderness
  and abdominal injuries, 90
  and bone injuries, 97, 98, 110
  and burns, 69
  and initial physical examination, 20, 21
  and internal bleeding, 54
  and muscle injuries, 108–9, 110
tetanus, 56
tingling in limbs, 83, 86
tongues, 39
transmission of diseases, 11–13
tuberculosis, 12, 14
tumours and seizures, 117

U

unconsciousness, 10, 79. *See also* responsiveness
unresponsiveness. *See* responsiveness

V

venous bleeding, 50, 60
vision changes, 10, 115
vomiting, 10
  and anaphylaxis, 64, 66
  and brain injuries, 79
  and internal bleeding, 54, 55, 59
  and poisoning, 125, 127
  and shock, 63, 66

W

weakness in limbs
  and brain injuries, 79
  and muscle injuries, 108–9
  and spinal injuries, 83, 86
  and strokes, 110, 115, 120
workplace and first aid, 3, 5
wounds
  and bone injuries, 97, 110
  care, 55–58, 59
  gaping, 10
  head wounds, 76–77, 78, 85
  open, 20, 21, 50–53, 55, 59
  puncture, 10

image credits

Chapter 1

Opener Courtesy of Larry Newell; 1-3 © Thomas M. Perkins/ShutterStock, Inc.

Chapter 3

Opener © Ingram Publishing/age fotostock;
3-2 © Jonathan Noden-Wilkinson/ShutterStock, Inc.

Chapter 4

Opener Courtesy of Larry Newell

Chapter 7

Opener, 7-2 Courtesy of AAOS.

Chapter 8

Opener © Joe Gough/ShutterStock, Inc.

Chapter 9

Opener © Gordon Swanson/ShutterStock, Inc.

Chapter 10

Opener © Cristoph & Friends/Das Fotoarchiv/Alamy Images

Chapter 12

Opener © Stockbyte/Creatas

Unless otherwise indicated, all photographs are under copyright of Jones and Bartlett Publishers, courtesy of the Maryland Institute of Emergency Medical Services Systems, or have been provided by the American Academy of Orthopaedic Surgeons.